Clinical communication skills

Edited by Peter Washer

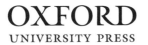

OXFORD

UNIVERSITY PRESS

OXFORD
UNIVERSITY PRESS

Great Clarendon Street, Oxford OX2 6DP

Oxford University Press is a department of the University of Oxford.
It furthers the University's objective of excellence in research, scholarship,
and education by publishing worldwide in

Oxford New York

Auckland Cape Town Dar es Salaam Hong Kong Karachi
Kuala Lumpur Madrid Melbourne Mexico City Nairobi
New Delhi Shanghai Taipei Toronto

With offices in

Argentina Austria Brazil Chile Czech Republic France Greece
Guatemala Hungary Italy Japan Poland Portugal Singapore
South Korea Switzerland Thailand Turkey Ukraine Vietnam

Oxford is a registered trade mark of Oxford University Press
in the UK and in certain other countries

Published in the United States
by Oxford University Press Inc., New York

British Library Cataloguing in Publication Data

Data available

Library of Congress Cataloging in Publication Data

Data available

Typeset in Swift by Graphicraft Limited, Hong Kong
Printed and bound
by L.E.G.O S.p.A, Italy

ISBN 978-0-19-9550463

Clinical communication skills

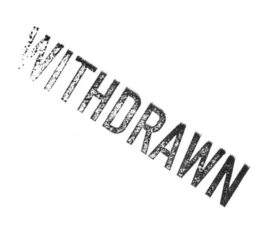

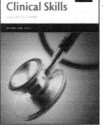
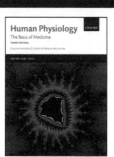
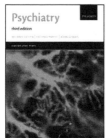
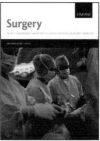
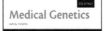
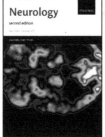

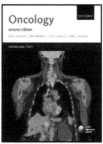
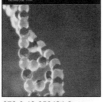
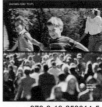
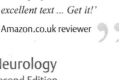

For Rowan Glenny

Preface

This book aims to bring together a range of evidence-based practical advice on the most effective ways to communicate with patients, families, and other professionals. It is primarily written for medical students, and spans their first contact with patients as students through to their early post-registration years as junior doctors.

Although the book's primary audience is medical students, I hope that the medical bias will not put off students of dentistry, nursing, social work, and professions allied to medicine, who will also find it useful reading. My original idea was to write a book for all students who have contact with patients, but in the end the danger was that it would become too general to be of use to anyone. Most of the communication challenges that face medics similarly face all health professionals, for example the issues around talking to children, to disabled people, to people from other cultures, and so on are the same. Even those parts of the book that are very medical-focused may still be relevant to other professionals. For example, although nurses do not take medical histories, it is nevertheless essential that they are able to read and understand medical notes.

Similarly, this book will be of value to post-registration health professionals; experienced doctors will find here the most recent research evidence on clinical communication. Although such research often finds its way into mainstream and specialist medical journals, much more is published in medical social science journals, where the average busy clinician may be unlikely to read it. Doctors trained before the introduction of a communication skills element to medical education will also find this book informative, particularly if their communication skills are to be assessed for the first time as part of their continuing professional development. Similarly those doctors trained in countries where communication skills are not formally taught will find this book offers a comprehensive introduction. Other post-registration health professionals, for example nurses moving into more specialist roles, will find that the later chapters in the book will help them to extend their communication skills into areas that may be unfamiliar to them, such as communicating risk.

I hope also that academics and clinical teachers will use this book to support their communication skills teaching. This book comprehensively surveys the field of clinical communication, but does not introduce any new theories or propose any new models. It could therefore be used either as a sole text or to complement other communication skills models and texts. The content spans the undergraduate clinical communication curriculum and is benchmarked against several international statements on doctor–patient communication, including the Toronto Consensus Statement (Simpson *et al.*, 1991), the Kalamazoo Consensus Statement (Makoul, 2001), the Royal Society of Medicine (RSM Forum on Communication in Healthcare, 2004), and the UK Council of Clinical Communication Teaching in Undergraduate Medical Education (von Fragstein *et al.*, 2008).

Finally, scholars may also find the Online Resource Centre associated with this book particularly convenient as a starting point for further research. They will find there both the *PubMed* references and full text links (where available) for all of the research papers used in writing the book, as well as web links to further reading from relevant charities, and international government and non-governmental organizations' reports.

Given the subject matter, I particularly wanted to have some element of patient and service-user involvement in the book, as well as a range of professional views. Therefore, during the course of writing it, I conducted a series of interviews with patients, relatives, and doctors. The resulting short recordings of these interviews are available to listen to as podcasts via the Online Resource Centre, and extracts from the transcripts of those interviews are used throughout the book. Patients are the real experts on doctors' communication skills, and their input illustrates the best practice points much better than I possibly could.

The book is written with an international audience in mind, and the research evidence used here comes from all over Europe, Australasia, and North America. That research shows that doctors and medical students face similar issues internationally. Having said that, it would be impossible to write from some God-like position outside of one's own culture, so foreign readers are asked to forgive any British cultural bias they perceive. In terms of use of language, for the sake of consistency, terms more common in Britain such as 'general practice' or 'general practitioner' have been used rather than 'Family Practice' and so on. In the UK education system, 'evaluation' means student feedback on a course, rather than a judgement of students' work,

so 'assessment' is used here to mean formative and summative assessments of students' work. Readers in North America are also asked to forgive the British English spellings.

I have enjoyed the challenge of writing and editing this book immensely and I do hope that readers will share my enthusiasm and enjoy reading it and learning from it. I am very open to being challenged and corrected, so please do get in touch with me (via the Online Resource Centre) with any feedback you have or any suggestions for future editions.

Peter Washer

References

Makoul, G. (2001). Essential elements of communication in medical encounters: The Kalamazoo consensus statement. *Academic Medicine*, **76**(4), 390–393.

RSM Forum on Communication in Healthcare (2004). Core curriculum for communication skills learning in medical schools. In: E. McDonald (Ed.), *Difficult Conversations in Medicine*. Oxford: Oxford University Press, pp. 209–211.

Simpson, M., Buckman, R., Stewart, M., Maguire, P., Lipkin, M., Novack, D., and Till, J. (1991). Doctor–patient communication: The Toronto consensus statement. *British Medical Journal*, **303**(6814), 1385–1387.

von Fragstein, M., Silverman, J., Cushing, A., Quilligan, S., Salisbury, H., and Wiskin, C. (2008). UK consensus statement on the content of communication curricula in undergraduate medical education. *Medical Education* **42**(11), 1100–1107.

Acknowledgements

I would like to thank the following people for their help and encouragement while writing and editing this book. Firstly, my partner Efisio, and all my friends and family, who have given me moral support over the past 2 years while this book has been in production. I owe a special debt of gratitude to my colleagues at Imperial College, London, for agreeing to allow me to disappear to Sardinia for the summer to finish the manuscript. I would like to thank Margaret Lloyd and Lorraine Noble, from whom I have learned so much, Shirley Cupit for putting me in touch with some of the people I interviewed for the podcasts, Katie Myers for her advice on smoking cessation, Jon Turney for generously giving his advice on the publishing process, and Caroline Connelly for her boundless enthusiasm. I am particularly grateful to all the people I interviewed for the podcasts, who gave me their time and shared their experiences. Some have used their real names and some pseudonyms, but they have all made this book much richer than it would otherwise have been. A special mention goes to all the students I have taught over the years and from whom I continue to learn so much. Finally, my thanks go to Shirley Cupit, Annie Cushing, Brian Douglas, Miriam Fine-Goulden, Linda Jones, Sukhmeet Panesar, Malcolm Thomas, Hazel Thornton, Jonathan Silverman, Susan Smith, Vivian Tang, and my anonymous reviewers, who read and offered their comments on early drafts. Their contributions have improved the book immeasurably. Any errors or omissions, as they say, are my own.

Contributors

Judith Cave is a consultant medical oncologist at Southampton General Hospital and St Mary's Hospital on the Isle of Wight.

Caroline Fertleman is a consultant general paediatrician at the Whittington Hospital in North London.

Melissa Gardner is a specialty registrar, in training to become a general practitioner.

Jayne Kavanagh teaches medical ethics and law at University College, London, and is also an associate specialist in sexual and reproductive health.

Simon Michaelson is a consultant psychiatrist at Northwick Park Hospital in North London.

Peter Washer teaches clinical communication at Imperial College, London.

Katherine Woolf is a research associate in medical education at University College, London.

Brief Contents

Detailed Contents

Introduction

Peter Washer

Previous generations of medical students were not taught clinical communication. Instead, people spoke of a doctor's 'bedside manner' – a personal attribute that they were lucky enough to be born with – or not – and certainly not something that could be taught (Suchman, 2003). Now, professional development has a place in the curriculum of most, if not all, medical schools, and this usually includes clinical communication, together with medical ethics, medical sociology, and public health (Stephenson *et al.*, 2001). This change in the medical curriculum has come about because the society in which medicine is being practised has changed, and because of a sense that the medical profession was becoming out of step with the expectations of patients. The background for this new book on clinical communication is thus the changing relationship between doctors, patients and their families, and other professionals.

One major change in the medical profession over the past few generations has been a move towards patient-centred medicine and away from doctor-centred, technology-centred, hospital-centred, and disease-centred medicine (Stewart, 2001). The term 'patient-centred medicine' was introduced by Balint (1964) and is an attempt to understand the patient's illness, and the symptoms and signs found by the doctor, not just in terms of the underlying disease, but also in terms of the patient's experience of their illness, and the impact of the illness on their lives (Henbest & Stewart, 1990). Patient-centred medicine seeks an integrated understanding of the patient's world, their emotional needs, and life issues, and aims to find common ground on the problem and its management (Stewart, 2001).

PODCAST

A professional perspective

"You were a medical student in the late 50s . . . In those days how did you learn how to talk with your patients?"

"Well, there was no such thing as learning communication skills; I'm not sure the phrase even existed at that time. Certainly amongst ourselves, amongst our fellow students, we talked: 'How do you talk to patients?' 'How do you get them to tell you what is wrong with them?' 'How do you put them at their ease?' And that was quite an important topic of conversation, which seemed less of a topic of conversation with our teachers. I suppose I learned by example, by having good role models – and some bad role models. Role models that I felt I very much wanted to imitate, I would like to be like them. And other people I felt, my goodness me, I really would like to avoid being like that particular person."

Podcast – Michael Modell, retired Professor of General Practice

Relationships between doctors and their patients used to be based on a 'doctor knows best' model of medical paternalism. Nowadays, patients increasingly want to share the process of making medical decisions with their doctors. This reflects a decline in deference to authority and hierarchy in Western society generally. Patients increasingly expect their own understanding about their experience of their illness, their preferences, values, and social circumstances to be taken into account (Coulter, 1999). This change coincides with the ability of patients to source medical information independently of their doctor via the Internet. In some cases, patients can rightly be said to be experts in their conditions, and this has led to the development of a new and more egalitarian relationship between doctors and at least some of their patients (Brown, 2008).

Another social trend that has impacted on the way medicine is practised has been an increasing sensitivity to the needs of minorities. Since the 1970s, there have been grass roots movements around the world arguing for equality and equal access to opportunities and services from a range of minority groups. Lesbian, gay, bisexual, and transgender people, disabled people, and people from ethnic minorities have all fought hard for changes in legislation and social attitudes to protect them from prejudice and discrimination. This lobbying has resulted in legislative changes in many countries, and this legislation is both influencing and reflecting changes in public perceptions.

There have also been changes in working practices within healthcare emanating from outside the medical profession, which have changed the way doctors work and have led to a greater emphasis on multidisciplinary team working. There has been an increasing, often resisted, culture of management and managerial scrutiny in healthcare. European legislation now limits doctors' working hours, and this has led to a reorganization of working patterns. Developments within nursing and other allied professions, such as new specialist nurse roles and other health practitioners, have led to a blurring of professional boundaries, with many roles that used to be the exclusive domain of doctors now fulfilled by other health professionals.

Finally, in recent years there has been a series of medical scandals that have shaken public confidence in the medical profession (Charles et al., 1999; Rosen & Dewar, 2004). In the UK in the 1990s, the so-called Bristol Babies scandal (Bristol Royal Infirmary Inquiry, 2001) found that 30 children had died unnecessarily as a result of cardiac surgery at the Bristol Royal Infirmary (Department of Health, 2002). In 2001, GP Dr Harold Shipman was found guilty of murdering 15 of his patients, although a subsequent enquiry estimated he may have killed up to 215 (Department of Health, 2005b). Also in 2001, what became known as The Three Inquiries were set up into four doctors: Dr Clifford Ayling, who was convicted of 12 counts of indecent assault against patients (Department of Health, 2004); Dr Richard Neale, who was banned from practising in Canada after the deaths of two of his patients as a result of his incompetence, yet continued to work, and raise concerns in the UK (Department of Health, 2004); and two consultant psychiatrists, Drs William Kerr and Michael Haslam, who were found guilty of sexual abuse of female patients (Department of Health, 2005a) having evaded numerous allegations made against them over the years, by discrediting their accusers and hiding behind their 'untouchable' status as consultants (Ehrich, 2006).

By the 1990s, the time was ripe for change in the medical profession. The profession proposed radical changes to the way doctors were trained and regulated. In the UK for example, the General Medical Council (1993) proposed devoting more attention to the teaching of clinical communication from the very start of training (Hargie et al., 1998), a move reflected around the same time in the USA (Association of American Medical Colleges, 1999), in Canada (Frank et al., 1996), and elsewhere.

This book reflects these changes to the medical profession and the medical curriculum and is written to support the learning and teaching of clinical communication at undergraduate level. The book starts with the basics of why we learn communication skills, with the process of a medical interview, and how to take a medical history. The middle section of the book covers how to talk with other professionals, to a diverse range of patients, to children and young people, and to people with mental health problems. The final section of the book covers the information-giving skills that junior doctors will need, including managing uncertainty, explaining risk to enable shared decision making, patient safety, dealing with complaints, and breaking bad news.

References

Association of American Medical Colleges (1999). *Contemporary Issues in Medicine: Communication in Medicine*. Washington DC: AAMC.

Balint, M. (1964). *The Doctor, his Patient and the Illness*. London: Pitman Medical.

Bristol Royal Infirmary Inquiry (2001). The Bristol Royal Infirmary Inquiry. London: HMSO.

Brown, J. (2008). How clinical communication has become a core part of medical education in the UK. *Medical Education*, **42**, 271–278.

Charles, C., Gafni, A., and Whelan, T. (1999). Decision-making in the physician–patient encounter: Revisiting the shared treatment decision-making model. *Social Science and Medicine*, **49**(5), 651–661.

Coulter, A. (1999). Paternalism or partnership? Patients have grown up – and there's no going back. *British Medical Journal*, **319**(7212), 719–720.

Department of Health (2002). *Learning from Bristol: the Department of Health's Response to the Report of the Public Inquiry into Children's Heart Surgery at the Bristol Royal Infirmary 1984–1995*. London: HMSO.

Department of Health (2004). *Committee of Inquiry – Independent Investigation into How the NHS Handled Allegations about the Conduct of Clifford Ayling*. London: HMSO.

Department of Health (2005a). *The Kerr / Haslam Inquiry: Full Report*. London: HMSO.

Department of Health (2005b). *The Shipman Inquiry: Independent Public Inquiry into the Issues Arising from the Case of Harold Frederick Shipman*. London: HMSO.

Ehrich, K. (2006). Telling cultures: 'Cultural' issues for staff reporting concerns about colleagues in the UK National Health Service. *Sociology of Health and Illness*, **28**(7), 903–926.

Frank, J., Jabbour, M., Tugwell, P., Boyd, D., Frechette, D., Labrosse, J., MacFayden, J., Marks, M., Neufield, V., Polson, A., Shea, B., Turnbull, J., and von Rosendaal, G. (1996). *Skills for the New Millennium: Report of the Societal Needs Working Group*. Ottawa: Royal College of Physicians and Surgeons of Canada.

General Medical Council (1993). *Tomorrow's Doctors*. London: GMC.

Hargie, O., Dickson, D., Boohan, M., and Hughes, K. (1998). A survey of communication skills training in UK schools of medicine: Present practices and prospective proposals. *Medical Education*, **32**, 25–34.

Henbest, R.J. and Stewart, M. (1990). Patient-centredness in the consultation. 1: A method of measurement. *Family Practice*, **6**(4), 249–253.

Rosen, R. and Dewar, S. (2004). *On Being a Doctor: Redefining Medical Professionalism for Better Patient Care*. London: Kings Fund.

Stephenson, A., Higgs, R., and Sugarman, J. (2001). Teaching professional development in medical schools. *The Lancet*, **357**, 867–870.

Stewart, M. (2001). Towards a global definition of patient centred care. *British Medical Journal*, **322**(7284), 444–445.

Suchman, A.L. (2003). Research on patient–clinician relationships: Celebrating success and identifying the next scope of work. *Journal of General Internal Medicine*, **18**(8), 677–678.

CHAPTER 1

Why learn communication skills?

Peter Washer

Learning points

This chapter will:

◆ explain the need to learn about clinical communication

◆ examine the evidence about how good doctors are at talking with patients

◆ assess the benefits of good communication for doctors . . .

◆ . . . and for patients.

Why do we need to learn about clinical communication?

'Why learn communication skills?' might seem like a strange title for an opening chapter of a textbook for medical students on communication skills. To be a doctor you need to learn about clinical sciences (anatomy, pharmacology, etc.) as well as clinical skills, such as examination skills. A textbook on anatomy or clinical skills would not need to start with a chapter entitled 'Why bother?' What's the point of learning communication skills when it's just talking, and you can do that already? Hopefully by the end of this chapter you will see that the reason you need to learn communication skills formally as part of a medical degree is because as good as your *general* communication skills may be, to be an effective doctor you need to learn effective *clinical* communication skills.

First I want to set you a task: Ask people you know about what their doctor is like, or ask someone who has recently been in hospital or had a loved one in hospital what the experience was like for them. Often patients will say that hospitals are noisy and that the food was awful, but generally the memories that people retain of their experiences of accessing healthcare are about the doctors and nurses they encountered. They will say, **'That doctor was so kind; she explained everything to me and I didn't feel I was rushed to make a decision'** or, **'Nothing was too much trouble for that nurse.'**

PODCAST

A relative's perspective

"Over the years you would have had a lot of experience of doctor's communication skills. In general what has been your impression?"

"In general we've been extremely fortunate. . . . They were wonderful human beings and they focused on our daughter and us as a family; and they gave us very helpful support . . ."

"Can I just go back to this question of them being wonderful human beings? How do you know they were wonderful human beings? Can we teach that to medical students?"

"You can, I am sure you can, yes. [laughs] Well, a concrete example, perhaps, is the professor at Great Ormond Street [children's hospital]. When we came into the room he would exclaim our daughter's name with such enthusiasm, as if she was the one person he most wanted to see, and he focused on her first."

Podcast – Catherine, mother of a daughter with Prader-Willi Syndrome

---

Analyse any patient enthusing about their experiences with healthcare professionals and most of the time you will find that the patient is talking about communication skills. Patients rarely say of their doctors: **'Her knowledge of pharmacology was the best'** or, **'His examination of my chest was amazing.'** Patients are not in a position to judge whether doctors are competent in these areas; they usually just assume, rightly, that doctors are experts and know what they are doing. However, the interface between that expertise and the patient's experience is the doctor's communication skills. From the patient's perspective, communication skills are what distinguish an excellent doctor (what you are hoping to become) from a merely competent one. Moreover, as we will see later in this chapter, doctors' poor communication skills are often at the root of patient discontent with healthcare, and are one of their principle motivations for complaints and litigation.

Generic communication skills for graduates

Good communication skills are important for people in all walks of professional life. If you were studying another degree instead of medicine, anything from computer science to drama to Spanish, your studies would also include learning communication skills, including how to produce written reports in a style appropriate to the discipline, how to engage effectively in discussions in a professional manner, how to do presentations, and how to communicate information, ideas, problems, and solutions to both specialist audiences and lay people. Some of these generic graduate communication skills will also form part of the subject of this book. In particular, in Chapter 4 there will be a discussion of the specific written communication skills you will need as doctors, and in Chapter 5 there will be a discussion of how to present information effectively in the context of medical practice.

'Medspeak'

Another aspect of communication that is common to all degrees is that students need to learn the professional jargon of the subject that they are studying. All professional groups – from engineers to philosophers – have their own jargon, and this jargon is mostly impenetrable to people outside their 'tribe'. Jargon is important and necessary, because it enables experts to communicate complex concepts to other experts in their field quickly and efficiently; it is a form of short-hand communication. The jargon that doctors use also marks out boundaries between themselves and lay people. As you become initiated into the medical 'tribe', you will learn to talk like a doctor. You also need to remember, however, that lay people will not understand 'medspeak'. At the same time that you learn the new language, you have to learn to do simultaneous translation back into everyday language when you talk to patients and their relatives. This applies not only to medical terminology, but also sometimes to everyday words and phrases, which often have different meanings for doctors and patients. For example:

When patients say:	they (usually) mean:
'sick'	generally unwell or in low spirits
'nerves'	depression or anxiety
'chronic'	really bad
'acute'	severe
'diet'	cutting calorie intake to lose weight
'drugs'	illegal drugs
'stomach'	abdomen
'history'	the study of the past
Whereas when doctors say:	**they mean:**
'sick'	vomit or vomiting
'chronic'	of long duration
'acute'	rapid onset
'diet'	what you eat
'drugs'	medicines
'history'	past illnesses
'firm'	a team of doctors and medical students
'shock'	life-threatening low blood flow
and so on.	

Beyond these generic writing and presenting communication skills, and the avoidance of using jargon (at least with patients), you will need to learn to gather information – to take a medical history – and explain and discuss medical diagnoses and treatments with patients.

The importance of the medical history in reaching a diagnosis

Making a diagnosis depends on three things:

- taking a medical history
- the physical examination of the patient
- the results of investigations carried out.

You might think that the investigations would be the most important of these three elements, yet, perhaps surprisingly, blood tests, X-rays, biopsies, ultrasound scans, three-dimensional imaging, and all the other clever ways that modern medical science has devised to look inside people's bodies often are not very useful until you know roughly what you are looking for. The medical history always was, and still is, the most important factor in reaching a diagnosis. Investigations are then useful to confirm or rule out what you already

suspect to be the case. For example, one UK study from the 1970s looked at how the diagnosis was established for 80 new patients presenting in a medical outpatients clinic. Doctors recorded their diagnosis after reading the patient's referral letter, after taking a history, and again after performing the physical examination. These diagnoses were compared with the diagnosis accepted 2 months later. In 66 out of 80 patients, correct diagnosis was made on the basis of the medical history alone (Hampton et al., 1975).

A generation later, a US study attempted to repeat the Hampton study. Doctors were asked to list their differential diagnoses for 80 medical outpatients with new or previously undiagnosed conditions and to rate their confidence in each diagnostic possibility after the history, the examination, and the laboratory investigation. Two months after the initial visit, the patients' records were reviewed to see what the accepted diagnosis was at that time. Although the physical examination and laboratory investigations were important in excluding certain diagnostic possibilities and increasing confidence in the doctors' diagnoses, in 61 out of 80 patients the diagnoses were still made from the clinical history (Peterson et al., 1992).

Effective clinical communication skills are thus an essential aspect of evidence-based healthcare. They are not something that can be bolted on once you have learned all the other things you need to learn to practise medicine. What used to be called a good 'bedside manner' is not something that you are born with – the research evidence shows that effective clinical communication skills *can* be learned and improved through training, and that this effect is lasting (Maguire et al., 1996b).

How good are doctors at talking with patients?

Are doctors not already good enough at talking with patients, without the need for formal training in communication skills? Unfortunately, research has identified systematic deficiencies in doctors' communication skills; for example, they routinely interrupt patients, redirect them, and do not let them finish giving their own story.

Doctors' early interruptions and redirections

Most medical consultations begin with the patient describing their complaint. The evidence shows that doctors often interrupt this description of the problem. For example, one North American study examined 264 interviews between general practitioners (GPs) and their patients and found that, while in 75% of cases doctors successfully solicited patient concerns, in 28% of the interviews, doctors redirected (interrupted) the patient's opening statement after a mean time of only 23 seconds. These interrupted opening statements were rarely completed. Nor were these interruptions particularly efficient, as those patients who were allowed to complete their statement of concerns used only 6 seconds more time on average than those who were redirected. In those interviews where doctors did not solicit the patient concerns during the interview, patients were more likely to raise further concerns later in the interview (Marvel *et al.*, 1999). Another US study of 60 GP visits found that patients spoke uninterrupted for an average of only 12 seconds after the doctor entered the room. A quarter of the time, doctors interrupted patients before they had finished speaking, interrupting them on average twice during a consultation (Rhoades *et al.*, 2001).

PODCAST

A professional perspective

"The most important thing I would say is do not appear rushed to the patient. An agitated doctor who is checking their watch or looking at the clock the whole time, or who appears distracted, will put the patient off. Once the patient has been put off they will lose confidence in you, and you will have to struggle hard to regain that confidence, if you are in fact successful. You may be very bright and very capable but when a colleague comes along, their patients will soon tell them: "Oh I didn't like that doctor; they didn't seem to have any time for me at all.""

 Podcast – Eileen Rosenfelder, GP

Soliciting the patient's 'real' agenda

The problem with redirecting patients early in the consultation is that the patients' 'real' agenda can be missed, and thus patients can leave the consultation with their reasons for visiting the doctor not having been addressed. Patients often have more than one concern, and even if they do have a single concern, it can be multifaceted, containing multiple medical, psychological, and social components. Patients often disclose their main concern only when they are about

to leave – the so-called 'by the way' syndrome, or 'door-knob concern' (Robinson, 2001).

Many patients leave their doctors feeling that their expectations of that visit have not been met. For example, one Californian study found that 11.6% of the 909 patients visiting their GP reported at least one unmet expectation. Patients who perceived an unmet expectation also reported less satisfaction with their visit, less improvement in their condition, and had weaker intentions to adhere to treatment plans. The doctors also rated those visits in which a patient had an unmet expectation as less satisfying and more difficult and demanding (Bell *et al.*, 2002). Another consequence of redirecting the patient from their own agenda is that doctors may not recognize those patients who are primarily seeking support rather than medical treatment. For example, a study of UK GP visits found that only four out of the 35 patients in the study voiced all their agendas in the consultation. The patients felt particularly unable to address:

◆ their psychosocial issues

◆ their worries about possible diagnoses and the future

◆ their own ideas about what was wrong with them

◆ their concerns about side effects, or not wanting a prescription

◆ information relating to the social context of their illness.

This often led to major misunderstandings, unwanted and/or unused prescriptions, and non-adherence (Barry *et al.*, 2000).

The benefits of good communication for doctors

Reducing stress and burnout

Having a doctor with excellent communication skills is clearly a benefit to patients (more about this below), but it is also beneficial to doctors themselves. As well as being uniquely rewarding, being a doctor and dealing with other people's life crises, with suffering, and with death can be very stressful and emotionally draining. Good communication skills can make you feel positive about your contribution to making some awful situations a little better. Conversely, if you feel you have not handled a situation well, then that can make you feel very bad about yourself. Developing your communication skills will help you be a better doctor for your patients, and will also help you enjoy your work.

As a professional group, doctors have very high levels of mental health problems and burnout (physical or emotional exhaustion caused by long-term stress). One study of 1133 UK hospital consultants found that around 27% of the consultants had evidence of mental health problems. Furthermore, they found that burnout was more prevalent among consultants who felt insufficiently trained in management and communication skills, with only half of them feeling that they had received adequate training in communication skills. The consultants were more likely to experience low personal accomplishment and high depersonalization (treating people in an unfeeling, impersonal way), to derive less stimulation from their job, and to have lower job satisfaction (Ramirez et al., 1996).

It is possible that another impact of doctors' poor communication may be to affect their ability to make the right clinical decisions. For example, one study of members of the American Society of Clinical Oncology indicated that those who had difficulty in communicating with their dying patients were more likely to see themselves as having failed those patients. This in turn was associated with a tendency for the oncologists to continue to prescribe chemotherapy in the terminal phase of illness (Mayer et al., 1998) (quoted in Baile et al., 1999).

Reducing complaints and litigation

The other benefit of good communication skills for doctors is the reduction in the amount of complaints and litigation, much of which relates to doctors' poor communication skills rather than to medical negligence or error. For example, one study analysed 227 patients and relatives who were taking legal action through five firms of (UK) medical negligence lawyers and found that the decision to take legal action was influenced not only by the original injury, but also by poor communication and the insensitive way the incident had been handled. Patients and relatives wanted to:

◆ prevent similar incidents happening to others in the future

◆ know how the injury happened and why

◆ hold the healthcare professionals or the organization to account for their actions

◆ gain compensation for the pain and suffering of the injury, or to provide for future care.

They wanted greater honesty, an appreciation of the severity of their trauma, and assurances that lessons had been learned. Even when compensation was vital, their motivation for litigation was not exclusively financial, but was determined by the original way the complaint was handled by the staff concerned (Vincent et al., 1994).

One fascinating US study found that surgeons who were more dominant and showed less concern and anxiety in their tone of voice were significantly more likely to have had malpractice claims made against them in the past. The authors audiotaped 114 conversations between 65 surgeons and patients, and 10-second extracts of these taped interviews were rated to assess the surgeons' warmth, hostility, dominance, and anxiety. The researchers found that they were able to predict accurately which of the surgeons had had malpractice claims against them from their communication skills ratings (Ambady et al., 2002). Evidence shows that a reduction in complaints and litigation can be achieved by training in communication skills (Lau, 2000).

The benefits of good communication for patients

Good communication skills are thus beneficial for doctors in that they have the potential to reduce stress and burnout, to limit the number of errors, and to minimize complaints and litigation. All of these factors are of course also beneficial to patients, but what of the more direct benefits of good communication to patients?

Effective communication and patient satisfaction

Research shows that patients judge consultations with their doctor to be positive when the doctor involves the patient in the management process. For example, one Swedish study of 46 GP consultations found that they were regarded as positive when:

◆ both GP and patient were in agreement about the reason for the consultation

◆ the GP asked about the patient's ideas, concerns, or health beliefs

◆ the GP took more time to explain and to achieve a shared understanding with the patient.

Interestingly, the positive consultations took no longer than the ones regarded as negative, despite the fact that the GP spent more time discussing the patient's concerns (Arborelius & Bremberg, 1992).

Effective communication and improved health outcomes

As well as increasing patient satisfaction, there is evidence that effective communication leads to improved health outcomes. For example, one Canadian study followed 272 patients presenting to their GPs with a new complaint of headache over a year. They found that when patients were asked about the number of headaches they had had in the previous month, about time lost from work due to headaches, and about any concerns they had about the headaches, the strongest predictor of resolution of headaches 1 year later was the patient's statement that they had been able to discuss their headache and the related problems fully with their doctor (The Headache Study Group of The University of Western Ontario, 1986).

PODCAST

A patient's perspective

"When the result arrived 8 weeks after, the doctor told me straightaway, a doctor I had never saw before, told me straightaway, 'You've got AIDS.' At that time there was no difference between HIV and AIDS, and they left the room to leave me to cope with this news. Of course I was feeling almost dead. I was giving myself 3 months to live, and 3 months after instead there I was, self-destructive, using more drugs and using more drink."

"What you're saying is that as a result of the test being handled really badly by the doctor's communication skills, you ended up getting even more self-destructive in the immediate period afterwards?"

"Yes. Nobody was asking me how I was feeling; it was only, 'Come to the hospital once a month to have a blood test and we'll tell you the answer next month when you come in.' But I don't know what the answer was, I don't know what they were looking for."

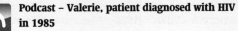 **Podcast – Valerie, patient diagnosed with HIV in 1985**

Research also shows that patients do better when they are provided with extra psychological interventions to help them deal with the medical crisis they are going through. For example, in one review of 34 studies in surgical or coronary care contexts, patients were split into two groups – one group that received more information or emotional support and a 'control' group who only received standard care. The review found that those patients who received enhanced communication input spent on average 2 days less in hospital than those in the control groups. This beneficial effect was despite the fact that most of the psychological interventions used were quite modest and in most studies were not matched in any way to patients' particular needs or coping styles (Mumford, Schlesinger & Glass, 1982).

Summary

Communication skills are an important component of clinical medicine. Although research shows that doctors' communication skills are often deficient, more positively, the research also shows that being a good communicator is something that can be learned and improved through training.

PODCAST

A professional perspective

"Did you feel that the communication skills you learned as a medical student were useful when you became a doctor?"

"Yes, I think that it suddenly became very evident why we were taught communication skills. I think that when it's the middle of the night and you haven't slept for many hours you are on auto-pilot, and you have actually at that stage to rely on the skills that are really deeply embedded in your brain and you are being taught. It comes as second nature to you, and you are suddenly thankful really."

Podcast – Kitty Mohan, recently qualified doctor

Poor clinical communication is often the source of patient dissatisfaction, non-adherence to treatment plans, medical errors, complaints, and litigation, and can lead to increased stress and rates of burnout in doctors. However, when doctors' communication skills are good, research shows that:

- complaints and litigation are reduced
- patients are more satisfied
- their health outcomes are improved.

The rest of this book will expand on these themes, and will talk you through what it means to be a good communicator in various contexts, giving you examples of different things you might say when faced with different and often difficult situations. Please do not think of these as the only 'right' way to respond – they are just suggestions. Instead, think of them as a toolkit of options that you can choose from to help prepare yourself for talking with patients, relatives, and other professionals in the years ahead. As you gain experience and mature as a professional, you will try out other ways of dealing with situations. Eventually you will develop your own style of communicating, your own professional voice, which will be authentic to your personality and tailored to the needs of your individual patients. This book will help you along that journey.

Further reading

Visit the Online Resource Centre for *Clinical Communication Skills* at: www.oxfordtextbooks.co.uk/orc/washer

References

Ambady, N., Laplante, D., Nguyen, T., Rosenthal, R., Chaumeton, N., and Levinson, W. (2002). Surgeons' tone of voice: A clue to malpractice history. *Surgery*, **132**(1), 5–9.

Arborelius, E. and Bremberg, S. (1992). What can doctors do to achieve a successful consultation? Videotaped interviews analysed by the 'consultation map' method. *Family Practice*, **9**(1), 61–67.

Baile, W.F., Kudelka, A.P., Beale, E.A., Glober, G.A., Myers, E.G., Greisinger, A.J., Bast, R.C., Jr., Goldstein, M.G., Novack, D., and Lenzi, R. (1999). Communication skills training in oncology. Description and preliminary outcomes of workshops on breaking bad news and managing patient reactions to illness. *Cancer*, **86**(5), 887–897.

Barry, C.A., Bradley, C.P., Britten, N., Stevenson, F.A., and Barber, N. (2000). Patients' unvoiced agendas in general practice consultations: Qualitative study. *British Medical Journal*, **320**(7244), 1246–1250.

Bell, R.A., Kravitz, R.L., Thom, D., Krupat, E., and Azari, R. (2002). Unmet expectations for care and the patient–physician relationship. *Journal of General Internal Medicine*, **17**(11), 817–824.

Hampton, J.R., Harrison, M.J., Mitchell, J.R., Prichard, J.S., and Seymour, C. (1975). Relative contributions of history-taking, physical examination, and laboratory investigation to diagnosis and management of medical outpatients. *British Medical Journal*, **2**(5969), 486–489.

Lau, F. (2000). Can communication skills workshops for emergency department doctors improve patient satisfaction? *Emergency Medicine Journal*, **17**(4), 251–253.

Maguire, P., Booth, K., Elliott, C., and Jones, B. (1996b). Helping health professionals involved in cancer care acquire key interviewing skills-the impact of workshops. *European Journal of Cancer*, **32A**(9), 1486–1489.

Marvel, M., Epstein, R., Flowers, K., and Beckham, H. (1999). Soliciting the patient's agenda: Have we improved? *Journal of the American Medical Association*, **281**(3), 283–287.

Mayer, R., Cassel, C., Emmanuel, E., and Schnipper, L. (1998). *Report of the Task Force on End of Life Issues*. 34th Annual Meeting of the American Society of Clinical Oncology, Los Angeles: ASCO.

Mumford, E., Schlesinger, H.J., and Glass, G.V. (1982). The effect of psychological intervention on recovery from surgery and heart attacks: An analysis of the literature. *American Journal of Public Health*, **72**(2), 141–151.

Peterson, M.C., Holbrook, J., VonHales, D., Smith, N.L., and Staker, L.V. (1992). Contributions of the history, physical examination and laboratory investigation in making medical diagnoses. *Western Journal of Medicine*, **156**(2), 163–165.

Ramirez, A., Graham, J., Richards, M., Cull, A., and Gregory, W. (1996). Mental health of hospital consultants: The effects of stress and satisfaction at work. *The Lancet*, **347**, 724–728.

Rhoades, D.R., McFarland, K.F., Finch, W.H., and Johnson, A.O. (2001). Speaking and interruptions during primary care office visits. *Family Medicine*, **33**(7), 528–532.

Robinson, J.D. (2001). Closing medical encounters: Two physician practices and their implications for the expression of patients' unstated concerns. *Social Science and Medicine*, **53**(5), 639–656.

The Headache Study Group of The University of Western Ontario (1986). Predictors of outcome in headache patients presenting to family physicians. A one year prospective study. *Headache: The Journal of Head and Face Pain*, **26**(6), 285–294.

Vincent, C., Young, A., and Phillips, A. (1994). Why do patients sue doctors? A study of patients and relatives taking legal action. *The Lancet*, **343**(8913), 1609–1613.

CHAPTER 2

The structure and process of the medical interview

Peter Washer

Learning points

This chapter will:

- describe how to introduce yourself and gain consent
- describe different questioning styles
- define empathy and explain how to demonstrate it
- illustrate ways to structure, check understanding, and close an interview.

From very early in your undergraduate studies you will start to meet patients and talk with them about various aspects of their health. As you progress, you will start to take more formal records of what they tell you to help your learning. Eventually, you will learn to take structured medical histories, initially to help your learning. Later, as you become integrated into the healthcare team, you will 'clerk' your own patients, for example when they are first admitted to hospital.

This chapter will talk you through the verbal and non-verbal communication skills required to interview patients. Chapter 3 will then describe in detail how to take a medical history and explain the content of that history, as well as give suggestions of ways to formulate questions in everyday language to gather all the information you need. Chapter 4 will describe how to subsequently write up a medical history, and Chapter 5 will describe how to present what you have discovered to your colleagues.

Introducing yourself and gaining consent

Setting the scene

Patients expect you to look the part, so always dress professionally and conservatively when you meet them. Casual clothes are likely to put patients off, and will make it more difficult for you to gain their trust and get their consent to speak to you. Another thing to think about before you approach a patient to interview them is the environment. Obviously you need to be able to see and hear each other clearly, particularly if the patient is elderly or has sensory impairments. Hospital patients often have a television or radio on at the side of their bed, so ask them if you can switch it off before you start talking. Interviews and examinations should ideally take place in an environment where they cannot be overhead or observed by other patients or visitors, and where you will not be interrupted. Close the door to the patient's room, or on open wards draw the curtains, which is sometimes the only privacy available. Put down any charts or paper while you are talking, and sit down and place yourself at about the same eye level as the patient. When doctors sit down, patients feel less rushed, and may even feel that the encounter lasts longer (Barnett, 2001). Sometimes in hospital wards there are no chairs available, but sitting on the bed can be interpreted as intrusive, and poses a cross-infection risk, so should be avoided. Finally, if you are also going to examine the patient, make sure you have all the right equipment or facilities before you start.

Introducing yourself and asking the patient's consent

When you introduce yourself to a patient, remember to use your full name and state that you are a junior doctor or a medical student and what year you are in. Avoid 'medspeak' – patients will not know what you mean if you say, **'I'm with Prof. Conway's firm'** or, **'I'm on my paeds rotation'** or, **'I'm an FY2 doctor.'** Get into the habit of saying: **'Hello, I'm Jasmeen Patel and I'm a first year medical student/junior doctor.'** Give the patient the warmest and most genuine smile you can muster – when you smile at someone, it is almost impossible for them not to smile back (try it!). If you judge it is appropriate, offer your hand to shake theirs, but remember some patients are more comfortable with shaking hands than others. Check the patient's name and their preferred form of address, but always assume

they are 'Mr . . .' or 'Mrs . . .' as a default option. Say, **'Can I just check your name? You're Mrs Susan Jones? Is it okay for me to call you Mrs Jones?'** If a patient wants you to use their first name, they will tell you so.

Then you need to set out why you want to talk to them and ask their permission to do so. If you are gathering information for your studies, then you need to say that you will be using their medical details to help you learn, and that you may write it up, but that whether or not they speak to you will not affect their treatment either way. Also, say that you will not use their names or any personal data that could identify them. If you are gathering information that will be used as part of their medical care, for example if you are taking a medical history that will be written into their notes, then you need to tell them that any information they give you will be confidentially held, but will be shared among the other members of the multidisciplinary team.

It is important to make this clear because often patients do not understand the difference between confidentiality and keeping secrets. In normal social circumstances, if a friend tells you a secret – for example someone tells you they have had an abortion – then they would expect that you would not pass on that information to anyone else under any circumstances. However, if a patient tells you that they have had an abortion in the past, then you will need to record that information in their notes, and it will be available to any other health professional who needs to know about it. If a patient starts to say, '. . . **I'm telling you this, but I don't want you to write it in my notes** . . .' then you need to stop them and remind them that, although what they say to you *is* confidential (to the healthcare team), you cannot keep it a secret. Of course, the other side of the coin is that you must *never* discuss confidential patient information outside of the healthcare team (or outside of the classroom if the patient has agreed you can use them as a case study), or indeed in any place where you can be overheard, such as in hospital lifts.

It is also useful to give patients some idea of how much of their time the interview will take. Then you need to ask their permission – to gain their consent – to interview them. You do not need to have this in writing, a verbal consent is sufficient. If for any reason a patient is not happy to go ahead, then you need to respect their wishes and accept that – they do not have to talk to you. Similarly, if at any point they change their mind, then they are at liberty to do so. When people are ill, tired, and stressed, they often do not want to talk, and you should not take it personally if they refuse. On the other hand, people in hospital or in waiting rooms are often bored, and talking to a friendly medical student can be a welcome distraction. If you follow the advice above and approach people sensitively and warmly, they will more often than not be very willing to help you.

Questioning styles

In the previous chapter, we discussed how research shows that doctors tend to interrupt patients before they have finished their opening narrative and therefore often miss important information, or do not let the patient reveal their full reasons for the visit (Marvel *et al.*, 1999). When you are talking to patients, rather than 'taking' a history from them, you need to think simultaneously about two narratives. One is from the patient's perspective – the illness from which they are suffering. The other is from the biomedical disease perspective, namely the signs (what you find on examining the patient) and the symptoms (what the patient tells you they are experiencing). Thus, you are engaged in a mutual conversation with the patient that includes both the biomedical disease perspective and the patient's experience of their illness (Haidet & Paterniti, 2003). Research shows that the most effective way to do this is by an appropriate choice of different questioning styles, usually starting with open questions and then moving on to closed questions to complete the picture and fill in any gaps in the information the patient has given you (Gafaranga & Britten, 2003; Maguire *et al.*, 1996a; Marvel *et al.*, 1999).

Open questions

Open questions are particularly useful for gaining wider knowledge or understanding and for finding out how people feel. They are used to encourage people to give information or to talk at length. Open questions often start with phrases like:

- '*Tell me* . . . what brought you into hospital?'

  or words like:

- '*What* . . . were you expecting from your visit to the doctor today?'
- '*How* . . . has the treatment been affecting you?'
- '*How* . . . are you getting on?'
- '*What's* been the trouble?'

'Why . . . ?' questions are best avoided, as they can sometimes seem threatening or judgemental, for example, '**Why do you smoke?**' A much more effective way of finding out the same information would be to ask, '**What usually triggers you craving a cigarette?**'

A reflective question is another type of open question, and can encourage people to elaborate on something they have already said. These mirror the other person's own words to encourage them to continue with their narrative. Reflecting a patient's words back to them also demonstrates that you have been listening to them. Examples might be:

- '**You say you have been worrying – in what way?**'
- '**You said you were frightened to talk to your wife about this. Can you tell me more about that?**'
- '**What do you mean when you say "drugs"?**'
- '**Confused? In what ways were you confused?**'

Or if a patient says, '**I was finding things getting more and more difficult**', you might reflect that back by saying, '**What sort of difficulties were you experiencing?**'

You should follow each open-ended question with a more focused open-ended question, for example, '**Tell me more about your headaches**'; and then once you have gathered all the information there is to gather about the headaches, ask the open-ended question: '**Do you have some other concerns?**' Ask this repeatedly until you have elicited their complete agenda. Then you can move on to closed questions to pick up any information that you need but that has not already been offered.

Closed questions

Closed questions are particularly useful for obtaining specific factual information or for confirming small pieces of information. The ways that closed questions are phrased suggest that a short, maybe one word, yes or no, answer is required. They are not generally helpful in promoting discussion or conversation around a topic, and so you should try to avoid overuse of closed questions, particularly early on in an interview. However, in certain circumstances, closed questions are essential. For example:

- '**Did you take your medication this morning?**'
- '**When was your last menstrual period?**'

They can also be particularly useful when discussing embarrassing topics such as when taking a sexual history. For example, asking: '**When was the last time you had sex . . . ?**', '**Was that with your regular partner . . . ?**', '**Did you use a condom . . . ?**' might be less embarrassing than asking: '**Tell me about the last time you had sex?**', which leaves the patient to decide which is the relevant information they need to disclose.

Checking questions are one type of closed question, used to confirm information. They are useful if you want to make sure you have understood correctly: For example, **'So your problem is with getting dressed. Is that right?'** or, **'So you've come to the doctor today for some contraceptive advice?'**

Students often try to gather all the information they need for a medical history through a series of closed questions, but this can turn into an interrogation; more questions can often mean less information gathered. This is not to say open questions are good and closed questions are bad. Rather, you will get the best result by appropriately combining the two.

Problematic question styles

There are some questioning styles that are particularly unhelpful and are probably best avoided altogether. Leading questions suggest an answer by the way they are phrased and imply that the other person will agree with you. Unfortunately, leading questions are often used by healthcare professionals, for example:

- **'You don't have a problem with that, do you?'**
- **'You'll agree that this is the best solution?'**
- **'You've taken the operation in your stride, haven't you?'**
- **'Are you feeling better today?'**

In particular, try to avoid talking in the first person plural: **'Are we feeling better today?'**, which suggests 'jollying the patient along', and practically forbids the answer: **'No, we're feeling a lot worse as a matter of fact!'**

Another problematic question style is stringing multiple questions into one complex sentence with many parts. This type of question can be confusing for a patient to answer, and similarly it can be confusing for you to interpret the answer they give you. For example, **'Do you think we've exhausted all the treatment options available now or do you think there's still a possibility that if we tried a new combination of medicines you might get some benefit?'**

Empathy and how to demonstrate it

Empathy is sometimes confused with sympathy, but empathy and sympathy are different. Feeling sympathy means that you share someone's pain, for example if a friend suffers a bereavement. This is possible even if you did not know the deceased; you feel pain because your bereaved friend does, and because you care about them. Empathy does not entail sharing the person's

pain in the same way. Having empathy means that we can project our feelings and thoughts, and emotionally identify with the other person's plight (Coulehan et al., 2001). Empathy means the human capacity to imagine what it might be like to be another person, to be in their situation, and therefore to understand how they feel.

Sometimes two types of empathy are distinguished:

- Cognitive empathy is a capacity to be aware of or to appreciate the viewpoints of others, particularly in regard to their motives, feelings, and need for help.
- Affective empathy is a tendency to react emotionally to the emotions of others, and is associated with warmth in interpersonal relationships (Munro et al., 2005).

Some patients' predicaments will naturally affect you more than others. Sometimes a patient will remind you of someone you love, or sometimes their circumstances are such that you find yourself getting more emotionally involved than usual. However, you do need to keep some level of professional distance between yourself and your patients. Patients are not your friends or family. What patients expect and need from doctors is medical advice and treatment, practical help, and emotional support and understanding. If you become too involved with your patients, there is a danger that you will become less able to provide what they need from you.

It is sometimes said that medical students start their training with a great deal of empathy and are motivated in their choice of career by a real desire to help other people. However, the experience of medical school can be brutalizing, and students learn to mask or deny their feelings, and to become detached. Students are taught to focus on diseases rather than patients, to talk about 'the case' rather than the person, and to be objective and impersonal. The purpose of studying medical humanities as part of your medical training is for you to understand more fully the experience of illness through novels, poetry, and art, and also to understand the effect that dealing with other people's suffering has on you. Reading and appreciating literature and art in medical humanities courses is intended to help you maintain or recover the empathy you very likely started your medical training with, and which sometimes gets lost along the way (Spiro, 1992).

You also need to communicate your empathy, and thus show that you understand the patient's perspective and feelings. We can demonstrate that we are empathic both verbally and non-verbally. Verbally, we might use phrases like:

- 'I can see how difficult this is for you.'
- 'I can tell you weren't expecting this news.'
- 'I'm really sorry you've had to go through this.'

Another type of empathic response is to validate the patient's reactions. For example:

- 'You really seem to have thought things through.'
- 'Most people in your situation would feel the same.'

Non-verbal communication

The other way we can demonstrate that we are empathic is through our non-verbal communication. Although non-verbal communication is sometimes viewed as a less critical aspect of medical care compared with what is actually said, research shows a strong association between doctors' non-verbal communication and patient satisfaction (Griffith *et al.*, 2003). For example, one US research project videotaped 36 GP interviews with patients. The doctors' non-verbal behaviour was rated by psychiatric nurses for various dimensions of rapport. Significant differences were found between the non-verbal behaviour of those doctors who gained high- and low-rapport ratings. Doctors were rated more positively if they sat directly facing the patient, with uncrossed legs, with both feet resting on the floor, with their arms in symmetrical, side-by-side positions, and if they engaged in moderate eye contact with patients. Low-rapport doctors tended to sit with their arms in asymmetrical positions, with one arm resting on a table or stand, to have their legs crossed and to be engaged in a greater or more extensive degree of eye contact (Harrigan *et al.*, 1985).

It is very important, therefore, to be attentive to the non-verbal signals you are sending. This includes:

- proximity, for example either facing the patient or placing your chair at a 90-degree angle
- nodding, smiling, looking interested, and making facilitatory noises, such as 'um hum'
- maintaining an open body posture, rather than closed. For example, folded arms signal wariness or hostility. Instead, signal attentiveness by leaning slightly forwards; upright or backward leaning postures may signal dominance or lack of concern. If you mirror the patient's body posture, for example by crossing your legs in the same way as they do, you are demonstrating that you are 'tuned in' and really listening to what they are saying
- holding eye contact appropriately, in order to demonstrate non-verbally that the patient is your main

focus. If you lose eye contact when a patient is telling you some crucial piece of information, for example to read their medical records, the patient may interpret the disengagement as signalling disinterest or disregard for their narrative (Ruusuvuori, 2001).

Having said all this, however, remember that too much or too little of these behaviours, for example holding eye contact for too long, can come across as over-familiar and thus have a negative effect. Therefore, you need to use your judgement in terms of what is appropriate, also bearing in mind the patient's age, ethnicity, and so on (Hall *et al.*, 1995). You can also use your body language to illustrate what you are saying, for example if a patient has just told you where their pain is, you can reflect this back to them by saying, 'So the pain starts here and moves down your arms . . .', at the same time using your hands to indicate on your own body where they have just told you the pain is.

Often students are unsure whether they are 'allowed' to touch patients, for example to comfort a patient who is upset. There can be no hard and fast rules regarding touch; you need to use your judgement as to whether it is appropriate or not, given both your and the patient's respective ages, genders, and cultural backgrounds. A general rule of thumb to guide you might be, if it feels right to touch a patient to show empathy, then it (probably) is right. Any touching is best kept brief and confined to the patient's more 'public' body surfaces – their hands, shoulders, and upper back (Hall *et al.*, 1995). If you have misjudged the situation, then you will soon pick that up from the patient's response and you can withdraw your hand.

One final aspect of non-verbal communication is the use of silence. Silence can be very powerful, although in Western cultures there is a tendency to feel uncomfortable with silences and to try to fill in gaps in conversations. Doctors who allow pauses in conversations without rushing in to fill them with questions or summaries will often collect additional information from their patients at key points simply by not speaking (Haidet & Paterniti, 2003).

Structuring, checking understanding, and ending the interview

Each medical interview should have a beginning, a middle, and an end. At the beginning, you introduce yourself, explain why you want to talk to the patient, and ask their consent. Then you ask about their problems and concerns using an appropriate balance of open and closed questions. After you have found all there is to know about each concern, you should summarize back to the patient what they have told you. This ensures that you have understood correctly, and it gives the patient an opportunity to add any other relevant information. For example:

'Can I just summarize what you've told me so far? You've told me that you've come along to the doctor's today because you've been suffering from constipation. For the past month or so you've only been going to the toilet once every 2 or 3 days, which is not normal for you, as you usually go every day. When you do go to the toilet it's quite painful, and your stools are hard but otherwise look normal. You don't have any idea why this should have happened, as you haven't changed your diet or anything. Otherwise you haven't noticed anything different or any changes in your health. You haven't tried any over-the-counter laxatives, and you're hoping the doctor can advise you and prescribe something that might help. Have I got that right?'

Then if the patient agrees with your account of what they have told you, you can signpost where you are in the consultation by saying: 'Okay, so far we've talked about your problem with constipation; apart from the constipation, is there something else you wanted from this visit today?' Usually doctors ask, 'Is there anything else?', but research suggests that this may be a leading question, which prevents patients disclosing any further expectations they might have. Although 'any' works in a question, you can't phrase a response with 'any' – for example: 'I have got any concerns'. One US study of 20 GPs randomly assigned 224 of their patients to be asked either, 'Is there anything else you want to address in the visit today?' or, 'Is there something else you want to address in the visit today?' They found that asking about 'something else' rather than 'anything else' eliminated 78% of unmet patient expectations (Heritage et al., 2007).

The patient may then introduce another concern or problem, and similarly you should explore that concern with an appropriate mix of open and closed questions. At the end of this process, again you do a mini-summary and ask if there is anything else. Research shows that asking about patients' additional concerns early in the visit, allowing them to talk without interrupting, addressing emotional and psychological issues, and exploring patients' beliefs and hidden agendas before you begin to close the interview decreases the likelihood that patients will introduce new problems late in the visit (White et al., 1997).

Incidentally, if during the course of a medical interview your mind goes blank, and you momentarily lose your train of thought and cannot think of what you are meant to say next, a brief summary is a useful way to get you and the patient back on track.

Once you have elicited all the patient's concerns, you can summarize their whole agenda back to them. Then you can signpost where you are in the interview by saying, 'Now you've told me about what's brought you along to the doctor's today, I'd like to ask you some other questions about your health. Is that okay?' If you are taking a full medical history, you can then move on from this part of the history – the presenting complaint(s) and history of the presenting complaint(s) – to the other aspects you need to cover. There is more about this in the next chapter.

While you are still a medical student, you must not give patients information or advice or offer a diagnosis, even if you know the information that they are asking you for. If a patient does ask you for information, say politely that you are a medical student so it is best if they ask a doctor or nurse, and tell them that you will ask a doctor or nurse to talk to them. When you are a junior doctor, before you close the interview you will need to give the patient information about what is wrong with them, discuss alternative courses of action, and involve the patient as much as they want to be in the decision-making process. Together you will then need to agree a plan of action, or at least summarize to the point that you have both reached, and outline what still needs to be agreed or done. The skills necessary for you to be able to do all this when you are a junior doctor are described in the final chapters of this book.

Ending the interview

Once you have gathered all the information you need, you can bring the interview to a close. Closure is the phase of the medical interview where you shift the focus from the present to what happens in the future. After your final summary, and (when you are a doctor) giving the patient information and forming a shared plan of action, it is important to say what happens next. This may simply be something like telling the patient they need to wait in the waiting room and the nurse will call them in for treatment, or that the doctor will see them as soon as possible, or it may be that they need to make another appointment to come back in 2 weeks. If at the end of the interview either you or the patient feels that the discussion has not been satisfactorily concluded, then you might need to make arrangements for another meeting or appointment.

Finally, once you have done all this, and before you leave the patient, always remember to say thank you.

Summary

Whether you are taking a full medical history, talking to a patient in a surgery or a ward before they see a doctor, or talking to a patient while you carry out some procedure, there are certain key communication skills that you should always use.

◆ Remember to introduce yourself properly, make it clear why you are talking to them and ask their permission to interview or examine them.

◆ Be attentive to the non-verbal signals you are sending.

◆ Use an appropriate mix of open and closed questions.

◆ Demonstrate empathy and understanding verbally and non-verbally.

◆ Check that you have understood the patient and that they have understood you by using signposting and mini-summaries as you go.

◆ Finally, summarize and close the interaction, making it clear what happens next.

These key communication skills should underpin *all* your interactions in *all* situations with *all* your patients.

Further reading

Maguire, P. and Pitceathly, C. (2002). Key communication skills and how to acquire them. *British Medical Journal*, **325**(7366), 697–700.

Although there are other clinical communication skills models, the most influential and widely taught is the Calgary-Cambridge Guide, outlined in:

Silverman, J., Kurtz, S., and Draper, J. (2005). *Skills for communicating with patients*, 2nd edn. Oxford: Radcliffe Medical Press.

There is also the useful Calgary-Cambridge website, the link to which can be found via the Online Resource Centre for Clinical Communication Skills *at:* www.oxfordtextbooks.co.uk/orc/washer

References

Barnett, P.B. (2001). Rapport and the hospitalist. *The American Journal of Medicine*, **111**(9B), 31S–35S.

Coulehan, J.L., Platt, F.W., Egener, B., Frankel, R., Lin, C.T., Lown, B., and Salazar, W.H. (2001). 'Let me see if I have this right . . .': Words that help build empathy. *Annals of Internal Medicine*, **135**(3), 221–227.

Gafaranga, J. and Britten, N. (2003). 'Fire away': The opening sequence in general practice consultations. *Family Practice*, **20**(3), 242–247.

Griffith, C.H., Wilson, J.F., Langer, S., and Haist, S.A. (2003). House staff nonverbal communication skills and standardized patient satisfaction. *Journal of General Internal Medicine*, **18**(3), 170–174.

Haidet, P. and Paterniti, D.A. (2003). 'Building' a history rather than 'taking' one: A perspective on information sharing during the medical interview. *Archives of Internal Medicine*, **163**(10), 1134–1140.

Hall, J.A., Harrigan, J.A., and Rosenthal, R. (1995). Non-verbal behaviour in clinician–patient interaction. *Applied and Preventive Psychology*, **4**(1), 21–35.

Harrigan, J.A., Oxman, T.E., and Rosenthal, R. (1985). Rapport expressed through non-verbal behaviour. *Journal of Nonverbal Behaviour*, **9**(2), 95–110.

Heritage, J., Robinson, J.D., Elliott, M.N., Beckett, M., and Wilkes, M. (2007). Reducing patients' unmet concerns in primary care: The difference one word can make. *Journal of General Internal Medicine*, **22**(10), 1429–1433.

Maguire, P., Faulkner, A., Booth, K., Elliott, C., and Hillier, V. (1996a). Helping cancer patients disclose their concerns. *European Journal of Cancer*, **32A**(1), 78–81.

Marvel, M., Epstein, R., Flowers, K., and Beckham, H. (1999). Soliciting the patient's agenda: Have we improved? *Journal of the American Medical Association*, **281**(3), 283–287.

Munro, D., Bore, M., and Powis, D. (2005). Personality factors in professional ethical behaviour: Studies of empathy and narcissism. *Australian Journal of Psychology*, **57**(1), 49–60.

Ruusuvuori, J. (2001). Looking means listening: Coordinating displays of engagement in doctor-patient interaction. *Social Science and Medicine*, **52**(7), 1093–1108.

Spiro, H. (1992). What is empathy and can it be taught? *Annals of Internal Medicine*, **116**(10), 843–846.

White, J.C., Rosson, C., Christensen, J., Hart, R., and Levinson, W. (1997). Wrapping things up: A qualitative analysis of the closing moments of the medical visit. *Patient Education and Counselling*, **30**(2), 155–165.

CHAPTER 3

How to take a medical history

Peter Washer

Learning points

This chapter will:

◆ describe how to take a medical history

◆ provide suggestions of ways to phrase the questions you need to ask in non-medical language

◆ discuss how to recognize and respond to a patient's cues.

Taking a medical history is a complicated business; in order to simplify it for learners, process and content are often taught separately. In medical school, you tend to learn about the process (how to do it), often using a communication model such as the Calgary–Cambridge model (Silverman *et al.*, 2005). Then, while on clinical placements, you focus more on the content of the medical history (what you need to cover), including the history of the presenting complaint, past medical history, social history, systems review, and so on. Unfortunately, this separation of process and content is, generally speaking, bad practice because it leaves many students with the impression that they are learning two entirely different models, rather than two aspects of the same thing (Kurtz *et al.*, 2003). It is difficult at first to remember to pay attention to both the process and content at the same time – it is a bit like that children's game where you have to pat your head with one hand and rub your stomach with the other and then swap hands.

To add to this complexity, communication skills are often taught separately from clinical skills such as examination skills, and procedural skills such as venepuncture or suturing. Of course, in real life medical practice, you need to be able to talk to patients *at the same time as* you are examining, taking blood from, or suturing them. One of the difficulties for learners is to fuse all these elements, including the clinical skills, the content of the history, the physical examination, the clinical investigations, diagnostic reasoning, and team working, and at the same time remember the underpinning communication skills (Kneebone & Nestel, 2005; Kneebone *et al.*, 2006). At the outset, it is best to separate all these things you need to learn and be as thorough as you can with each aspect. As you get more experienced, you will to start to knit all these elements together.

Taking a medical history

The medical history is a structured enquiry in which you need to find out about a number of different topics to make sure you have covered all the relevant ground. Each doctor has their own individual style of history taking, and this is something you'll grow into as you mature as a professional. The best advice when you start taking a patient's medical history is to begin by asking an open question. Then sit back, keep quiet, and listen for a good 2 or 3 minutes while the patient tells you just about everything you need to know. If you let patients tell their own stories in their own words, they will more often than not cover most of the information you require. The trick is to listen attentively, mentally tick off the information you need as they give it to you, and then go back and probe further for the things that they have not already told you.

All this is of course easier said than done, especially when you are starting out, but if you observe your seniors, you will see how the two narratives of the patient's perspective on the illness and the biomedical disease model can be fused. The patient's narrative will not come out in the sequence that you need to write it or present it (as described in Chapters 4 and 5), but it will be a fuller account of their symptoms, and the impact of those symptoms on their lives, than you could possibly elicit using a list of closed questions.

Once you have listened to the patient's narrative, you need to move on to the questions you will need to ask for the fuller picture. It is useful to signal to the patient that the questions that you are going to ask are 'normal' or standard, in case they get concerned that you are probing some area because you suspect something sinister is wrong with them. Finally, it is useful to signpost when you move from one topic to another, for example, '**Now I've asked you about the medicines you've been taking, I need to move on and ask you some questions about your family.**'

THE STRUCTURE OF A MEDICAL HISTORY

- The presenting complaint(s)
- The history of the presenting complaint(s)
- Past medical history
- Drug/allergy history
- Family medical history
- Personal and social history
- Systems review

Ways to phrase the questions in non-medical language

The first thing to be acutely aware of when taking a medical history is your use of jargon and medical terminology. You cannot assume that patients will know the meaning of even relatively everyday words like 'hypertension', or what pain 'radiating' means, let alone what dyspnoea is. Similarly, you cannot assume that a patient has understood just because they have not picked you up on some medical terminology you have used. Patients often either do not hear the medical word, or else they will try to make sense of it themselves from the context, often feeling that they should know what it means. Therefore, you should *always* translate 'medspeak' and medical jargon into everyday language. Suggestions of how you might phrase your questions in everyday language are included below. If a patient does use a medical word like 'palpitations', ask them to describe what they mean so you are clear that you mutually understand each other.

Another thing that can cause students difficulties is that it can be hard to keep the person 'on topic', and it is difficult to interrupt without seeming rude. If a patient's narrative seems to be rambling and unfocused, then wait until they pause – even the most garrulous patient has to take a breath at some point – and do a mini-summary of the interesting points of what they have told you so far. Ask them, **'Have I got that right?'** Then the patient can elaborate or not, and following that, you should be able to re-focus them by saying, **'I just need to ask you some more questions about . . .'**

The usual abbreviations for the various subheadings of the medical history are included here. There is more on these abbreviations in the next chapter.

The presenting complaint(s) (PC)

The first task in a medical history is to define the problem(s) that are troubling the patient. This is known as the 'presenting complaint' although it is more properly the 'patient's problems'. You do this by asking an open question like:

- **'Can you tell me about why you've come to the doctors today?'**

- **'What brought you into hospital?'**

For example, a patient might be admitted to hospital complaining of severe 'stomach' pain. When you ask them what the problem is, they might say, that apart from the pain, they think they have lost quite a bit of weight. You record that as:

PC

1 Abdominal pain

2 Weight loss

The history of the presenting complaint (HPC)

In order to evaluate the presenting complaint(s), you need to find out more information about it. There are two aspects to this: one is to explore the medical (disease) perspective of the signs and symptoms and to look for clues that will lead you to a diagnosis. The other is to explore the patient's perspective on their illness, and find out how it affects them, as well as their ideas about it.

The medical (disease) perspective

Sequence of events:

- **'When were you last well?'**

- **'How long have you had the problem?'**

Symptom analysis:

- **'Can you tell me which part of your body is affected?'**

If patients are complaining of pain, try to avoid leading questions, such as, **'Does exercise bring the chest pain on?'** Instead, use the so-called 'pain sieve', the common mnemonic used is SOCRATES:

Site
- **'Can you tell me or show me where the pain is?'**

Onset
- **'Have you ever experienced this type of pain before?'**
- **'When does it come on?'**

Character
- **'Can you describe the pain in your own words?'** (If you give patients a list of adjectives: 'stabbing', 'throbbing', and so on, they will inevitably choose from that list.)

Radiation
- **'Does the pain go anywhere else?'**

Alleviating factors/associated symptoms
- **'What do you do about it when it happens?'** or, **'Have you tried anything to make it better? Did that help?'**
- **'Is there anything else associated with the pain?'**

Timing

- ◆ 'Is the pain constant or does it come and go?'
- ◆ 'How long does it last?'

Exacerbating factors

- ◆ 'Does anything make it worse?'

Severity

- ◆ 'How painful would you say it is on a scale of one to ten?'

The patient's (illness) perspective

As well as the biomedical signs and symptoms, you need to explore the patient's perspective about their experience of their illness. Most patients will have their own thoughts and worries about what is wrong with them, and what they possibly need to help them get better. For example, one UK study of 756 patients attending GP appointments found that most patients came to the consultation with a particular agenda. Almost all of them had treatment or investigation requests they wanted to make of the doctor, 40% consulted the doctor because they had become concerned about their symptoms, and 60% had their own ideas about what was wrong (McKinley & Middleton, 1999). One easy formula to remember is to ask them about their own ideas, concerns, and expectations (Tate, 2005) – this is often shortened to the acronym ICE:

Ideas (their thoughts about what might be the nature and cause of the problem)

- ◆ 'Have you got a view on what might be causing this problem?'

Concerns (anxieties relating to the seriousness or implications of the problem)

- ◆ 'Do you have any particular worries about what could be wrong?'

Expectations (the doctor's likely reaction)

- ◆ 'What were you hoping for from this visit to the doctor today?'

Another aspect of the patient's experience of their illness that you need to explore is how it affects their daily life:

- ◆ 'How does this affect a typical day?'

Remember to ask if the patient has other expectations or concerns that they want to raise after you have found out about the presenting complaint.

Past medical history (PMH)

Once you have explored the history of the presenting complaint and the patient's ideas, concerns, and expectations, you need to fill in the background information to give some context for the presenting complaint.

IMPORTANT COMMON CONDITIONS TO BEAR IN MIND

While you should avoid interrogating the patient with a series of closed questions right away, at the same time there are some important common conditions that you need to rule out. You need to find out whether the patient has suffered from the following:

The acronym THREADS J is useful to ensure you have not missed anything:

Tuberculosis
High blood pressure/heart attack/heart disease
Rheumatic fever
Epilepsy
Asthma/anaesthetic problems
Diabetes
Stroke
Jaundice

A useful way to start finding out about the patient's past medical history is to ask broad questions. These will direct you to more targeted questions if you get a positive response:

- ◆ 'Do you suffer with any long-term medical conditions?'
- ◆ 'Have you had any illnesses or been in hospital in the past?'
- ◆ 'Have you had any operations?'

If these broad questions and any subsequent follow-up questions still have not covered some of the common conditions in the list above, then ask closed questions to make sure you have not missed the outstanding ones.

Drug history (DH)

Before adjusting medications or considering prescribing anything new, doctors need to know what the patient is already taking. If the patient has brought their medicine containers with them, then go through them one by one and check these together with the patient. Whether or not they have brought their current medication with them, you need to ask:

* 'Are you taking any medicines, tablets, drops, or inhalers?' (Avoid the word 'drugs', which for most people means illegal drugs.)

* 'Do you know what doses you take?'

* 'Do you manage to take them regularly?'

* 'Do you remember whether you've taken any other medicines in the past that you're not taking now?'

* 'Are you taking anything else, such as over-the-counter medicines or complementary medicines?' (See Chapter 12 in this book for a further discussion of the importance of asking about complementary and alternative medicines.)

* 'Are you allergic to anything you know of?'

Family medical history (FH)

Next you need to ask about the patient's family's medical history, particularly their first-degree relatives – parents, siblings, and children. You will need to tailor these questions depending on the patient, so for example it might not be appropriate to ask a very elderly patient if their parents are still alive. You will need to ask about the family medical history in more detail if what is wrong may have a genetic component. When asking about first-degree relatives, you should be aware that some people may have no contact with or information about any blood relatives, for example people who are adopted. Ask:

* 'Are your parents alive?' and if so, 'Are they well?'

* 'Do you have brothers or sisters? Are they well?'

* 'Did any of these close relatives die young? If so, how?'

* 'Do any of your relatives suffer with illnesses that might run in the family?'

Personal and social history (SH)

Under this heading, you need to ask some sensitive questions to explore the patient's home circumstances. Use language carefully here, as you do not want to exclude any possibilities, for example separated or divorced couples still sharing a home, lesbian or gay partners, (platonic) room-mates, and so on. Ask a catch-all question to investigate the patient's living arrangements and relationships such as:

* 'Who's at home with you?' You may need to follow this up with more questions, including asking about deaths, estrangements, and divorce, such as 'Have you been widowed long?' 'Do you have family living close by?'

* 'What do your friends and family think about what is wrong with you?'

If appropriate given the age and health status of the patient, you will need to ask, some of the following questions:

* 'Do you manage to do your own shopping and housework?' If not, ask, 'What help do you get?'

* 'Do you need any other help at home?' Again you might need to follow this question with more questions to investigate whether or not the patient manages to wash themselves and go to the toilet unaided, or whether they have contact with community nurses or home care services.

* 'Do you work? What job do you do? Do you enjoy it?' or 'What job did you used to do?'

It is important also to ask about risk factors. If people do indicate that they have risk factors for ill health and would like to change their behaviour, remember to at least flag up at this point the possibility of health promotion advice, or mention what support is available, for example referral to a dietician or smoking cessation specialist. Ask:

* 'Are you a current smoker?'
  o If not, ask if they have ever smoked. If yes, ask how many a day, for how long, and when they stopped.
  o If yes, ask how many cigarettes they smoke a day, and how long they have smoked. *Always* enquire if they have thought about stopping.

* 'Do you drink alcohol? If so, how much do you drink and how often?'
  o Record this in terms of units of alcohol per week: one unit is half a pint or 50 ml of beer, 25 ml of spirit (most bars serve 35 ml) or 80 ml of wine (a small glass). If they reveal that they are regularly drinking more than the recommended amounts (3–4 units a day for men, 2–3 units a day for women), then you should explore further to detect hazardous drinking or alcohol dependence (see Chapter 11 for more information on alcohol screening questions).

- (If appropriate) **'Do you use any recreational drugs?'**
- **'What sort of food do you eat? Talk me through what you eat on a typical day.'**
- **'Do you do any physical exercise or sport?'**

Systems review/systems enquiry (SE)/ systematic questions (SQ)

In the last part of the medical history, you need to run through a list of major common symptoms of each body system, although you do not need to repeat any questions that have already been answered fully. This is a final 'belt and braces' check in case the patient has been experiencing symptoms that they have not told you about already, particularly symptoms that may be associated with their presenting complaints(s) but which they have not thought themselves may be connected.

General health

- **'Apart from what you've already told me about, are you generally well?'**
- **'Do you have enough energy or do you find you get tired during the day?'**
- **'Do you sleep well?'**
- **'How's your appetite?'**
- **'Do you ever get a fever or have sweats at night?'**
- **'Is your weight stable?'** or, **'Has your weight gone up or down recently?'**
- **'Do you have any problems with your skin such as rashes or bruises?'**
- **'Have you got any sore areas where you've been sitting or lying?'** (pressure sores).

Cardiovascular system (CVS)

- **'Do you ever get pain in your chest?'** If so, explore using the SOCRATES mnemonic above.
- **'Do you ever get short of breath?'** If so explore whether this is during exercise or at rest, at night (paroxysmal nocturnal dyspnoea) or when they lie down (orthopnoea).
- **'How far would you say you can walk before you get tired?'** (exercise tolerance).
- **'Does your heart ever beat very fast, or feel like it's pounding in your chest?'** (palpitations).
- **'Do you get pain in your calves when you walk?'** (claudication).
- **'Do your ankles get swollen?'** (oedema).

Respiratory system (RS)

- **'Do you wheeze or have a cough?'** If so, **'Does it hurt when you cough?'**
- **'Do you ever cough anything up?'** (sputum – they might use the word 'phlegm') and if so, **'What colour is it?'** and **'Is there any blood in it?'**

Gastrointestinal system (GI or GIS)

- **'Do you ever get any abdominal pain?'** If so, explore using the SOCRATES mnemonic.
- **'Do you ever feel sick or vomit?'** If so, **'Is there any blood in your vomit?'**
- **'Do you have any problems chewing or swallowing?'**
- **'Do you get indigestion or a burning pain in your chest after eating?'** (heartburn).
- **'Do you open your bowels regularly?'**
- **'Have there been any changes in your bowel habits recently?'**
- **'Can you describe the colour and consistency of your stools?'**

Genitourinary system (GU)/gynaecological

- **'Do you have any difficulty passing water?'** If so, explore whether they suffer from incontinence, poor stream, dribbling, or pain on passing urine
- **'Do you have to pass water frequently?'** If so, **'Do you have to get up during the night to go to the toilet?'**
- **'What colour is your urine?'** **'Is there ever any blood in it?'**
- **'Do you have a sexual partner?'** If so, **'Do you have any problems with your sexual relationship?'**
- **'Do you have any discharge (from your penis or vagina)?'**
- For all women:
  - **'At what age did your periods start?'**
  - **'Have you ever been pregnant?'**
- For pre-menopausal women,
  - **'Are your periods regular?'**
  - **'How heavy would you say they are and how long do they last?'**
  - **'Is there a possibility you could be pregnant now?'**
- For post-menopausal women,
  - **'When did you have the menopause?'**
  - **'Do you ever have any vaginal bleeding?'**

Central nervous system (CNS) or neurological system (NS)

+ 'Do you get headaches or migraines?'

+ 'Have you ever had any fits or fainting or "funny turns"?'

+ 'Do you ever get any tingling, pins and needles, or numbness anywhere?'

+ 'Do you suffer from any weakness in your arms or legs?'

+ 'Do you have any problems with your eyes or your vision?' (disturbances).

+ 'Can you hear well?' and 'Do you ever get ringing in your ears?' (tinnitus).

+ 'Have you noticed if you have any problems speaking?'

+ Psychiatric –
  ○ 'How is your mood? Do you ever feel down or depressed?' If so, explore whether there are any changes in their appetite or sleep patterns, such as waking early, or if they get tearful.
  ○ 'Have you noticed any changes in your ability to remember things?'
  ○ 'Do you get very anxious or stressed?' (Patients will sometimes talk about having 'bad nerves', which usually means anxiety.)

Musculoskeletal system

+ 'Do you suffer from any muscle pain or weakness?'

+ 'Do you get pains or stiffness or swelling in your joints?'

Endocrine system

+ 'Do you suffer when it's very hot or cold?' (intolerance)

+ 'Do you find you sweat more than usual?'

+ 'Do you ever get very thirsty?'

Recognizing and responding to cues

Sometimes the patient's meaning or the substance of their concerns is hidden beneath the content of what they are saying. You need to look out for, and respond to, any cues that they might be giving you. In the course of taking a medical history, they might make a 'throwaway' comment that seems unrelated to what you are talking about at that time, or they might hesitate at some crucial moment, or might describe something using particularly strong language, or using an odd turn of phrase or metaphor. Despite your best efforts at eliciting all their concerns early on, another way that patients' real concerns surface is at the end of the interview, the 'while I'm here doctor' or so-called 'by the way . . .' or 'doorknob' syndrome. A rambling history often conceals a hidden agenda.

In the previous chapter, the importance of attending to the non-verbal signals that you are sending out was stressed, but of course this works in both directions. The patient's non-verbal communication can reveal the emotional impact of their illness and can thus be diagnostically useful (Hall *et al.*, 1995). One way that patients will cue that there is something else troubling them is through non-verbal signals. They might lose eye contact or look down at a crucial point, avoid a question, or become quiet and distant. Research shows that, while doctors respond well to cues for medical information, emotional cues are handled less well. For example, one Australian study of 298 consultations between cancer patients and oncologists found that two-thirds of the patients' cues concerned medical information, which the doctors effectively identified and responded to. However, the older and male patients, particularly, gave significantly fewer emotional cues, were reluctant to disclose emotional concerns, and asked fewer questions; and doctors were less observant of and able to address those cues for emotional support (Butow *et al.*, 2002).

If you do notice a patient's cue, let the patient finish what they are saying and then go back and follow it up. Be transparent that you have noticed something and you want to give them the opportunity to talk about it further. For example, you might say: '**When you were telling me about your family earlier, I noticed you seemed very quiet and looked a bit upset by my question. Was there any particular reason for that, or was there something else you wanted to talk about?**'

One aspect of patients' non-verbal behaviour that is particularly diagnostically useful is their facial expressions of pain. A review of research on the facial expression of pain found that observers tend to underrate pain based on facial expression, so you need to be aware of this bias and take it into account when trying to evaluate how much pain a patient is suffering. If you can see from a patient's facial expression that they are in pain, the chances are that, from the sufferer's point of view, the pain is intense. On the other hand, the absence of a facial expression cannot be interpreted as indicating that there is no pain (Prkachin & Craig, 1995).

Summary

A medical history is structured in such a way that nothing is missed and is written up in a standard format so that any other health professional can easily locate a relevant piece of information they might need.

Learning to take a full medical history can be daunting, and equally from the patient's perspective there is a lot of information exchanged. Sometimes it is only possible to take parts of the history at a time, for example in emergency situations or when a patient is in pain, confused, or generally too unwell. Remember that, although you have to collect all this information to reach a diagnosis, the problems that you might think medically are the most important may well not be the patient's priorities. Attend to the patient's narrative first and follow their agenda, filling in all the other information you need after you have listened closely to their story. As William Osler famously said: *'Listen to the patient . . . they are telling you the diagnosis.'*

Further reading

The medical history is part of the consultation, and is followed by an examination of the patient. The most comprehensive and student-friendly book on examination and clinical skills is:

Cox, L.T. and Roper, T.A. (2005). *Clinical Skills*. Oxford: Oxford University Press.

Visit the Online Resource Centre for *Clinical Communication Skills* at: www.oxfordtextbooks.co.uk/orc/washer

References

Butow, P.N., Brown, R.F., Cogar, S., Tattersall, M.H., and Dunn, S.M. (2002). Oncologists' reactions to cancer patients' verbal cues. *Psychooncology*, **11**(1), 47–58.

Hall, J.A., Harrigan, J.A., and Rosenthal, R. (1995). Non-verbal behaviour in clinician–patient interaction. *Applied and Preventive Psychology*, **4**(1), 21–35.

Kneebone, R. and Nestel, D. (2005). Learning clinical skills – The place of feedback and simulation. *The Clinical Teacher*, **2**(2), 86–90.

Kneebone, R., Nestel, D., Yadollah, F., Brown, R., Nolan, C., Durack, J., Brenton, H., Moulton, C., Archer, J., and Darzi, A. (2006). Assessing procedural skills in context: Exploring the feasibility of an Integrated Procedural Performance Instrument (IPPI). *Medical Education*, **40**, 1105–1114.

Kurtz, S., Silverman, J., Benson, J., and Draper, J. (2003). Marrying content and process in clinical method teaching: Enhancing the Calgary–Cambridge guides. *Academic Medicine*, **78**(8), 802–809.

McKinley, R.K. and Middleton, J.F. (1999). What do patients want from doctors? Content analysis of written patient agendas for the consultation. *British Journal of General Practice*, **49**(447), 796–800.

Prkachin, K. and Craig, K. (1995). Expressing pain: The communication and interpretation of facial pain signals. *Journal of Nonverbal Behaviour*, **19**(4), 191–205.

Silverman, J., Kurtz, S., and Draper, J. (2005). *Skills for Communicating with Patients*, 2nd edn. Oxford: Radcliffe Medical Press.

Tate, P. (2005). Ideas, concerns and expectations. *Medicine*, **33**(2), 26–27.

CHAPTER 4

Writing about patients

Peter Washer

Learning points

This chapter will:

◆ provide some best practice guidelines to follow when writing about patients

◆ explain how to write up a medical history

◆ identify and discuss other forms of written medical communication.

Like all professionals, doctors need to be able to communicate effectively in writing and to be able to give presentations. This chapter will explain how to write up a medical history, before examining some other forms of communication between doctors, patients, and other health professionals.

Best practice in written medical communication

The 'case notes', or 'case records', are the record of the patient's care, and these may be recorded and stored in handwritten or electronic form. Keeping accurate case records is an essential aspect of medicine, especially when a range of different doctors and other healthcare professionals may be involved in a particular patient's care. Case records are usually shared among members of the multidisciplinary team (MDT) and with other teams; therefore the patient's notes should include sufficient detail for the consultation or patient contact to be mentally reconstructed, and thus enable a seamless continuity of patient care (Medical Protection Society, 2008).

Always bear in mind that patients, relatives, and their representatives are entitled to see their medical records, a principle established in UK law by the Access to Health Records Act 1990 and the Data Protection Act 1998. In the event of a complaint, a claim for compensation, or disciplinary action, records will be used as legal evidence. Therefore, they should always be clear, objective, contemporaneous, tamper-proof, and original (Medical Protection Society, 2008). Whenever you write anything down about a patient, always err on the side of caution. Imagine reading it out loud to the patient, their family, or in a worst-case scenario, to a Coroner's Court. If you would feel uncomfortable doing so, that is a good indication that you need to reconsider what you are about to write.

At the same time, remember that the patient's record is also a record of the intellectual process of your diagnostic reasoning and management plan, and can therefore protect you if things go wrong. Even if, in hindsight, you got the diagnosis wrong or made the wrong management decisions, you will still be able to use the patient's notes to demonstrate retrospectively what you found on the basis of the history and examination, and why you reached the conclusions you did at the time, and to justify the management decisions you made.

Some points to remember are:

- Notes that you intend to take off the ward or out of the clinic or surgery can get lost or stolen. If this happens, patient information should not be compromised. Therefore, if the purpose of your note taking is your learning, rather than making notes that will become part of the patient's record, you should not write down any information that might identify the patient.

- Anything you write in the patient's record should be clear and legible. Illegible handwriting poses a threat to patient safety, particularly in relation to prescriptions. For example, a man suffered irreversible brain damage after a pharmacist misread his doctor's badly written prescription for the antibiotic Amoxil® (amoxicillin) for a chest infection, as Daonil® (glibenclamide), a drug used to lower blood sugar in people with diabetes. As a result of taking the wrong medicine, the patient went into a coma and was hospitalized for 5 months, suffering blunted intellect and poor short-term memory as a result (Department of Health, 2002).

- Always use an indelible black ballpoint pen, as other colours do not photocopy well, and fountain pens can leak or be difficult to read.

- Each entry made in the patient's record should have clearly written next to it: your name, with your surname printed in capital letters, your position (for example 'fourth-year medical student'), the date, and your signature. If you make any alterations later, for example to correct a mistake, the amendment should be similarly signed and dated, so that it is clear you have not tried to tamper with the notes in an attempt to deceive anyone.

- Each page of a patient's notes should be numbered consecutively, and should have the patient's name and hospital or patient number or bar code sticker on it.

How to write up a medical history

When you assess the patient, the notes that you write up are called 'patient clerking', and include a record of the medical history you have taken, the examination you have carried out, your findings, a list of what you think the diagnosis or diagnoses could be, and what you propose as a management plan.

Although writing at the same time as you are talking and listening to the patient is often criticized as being distracting to the patient, in effect it is almost impossible to remember everything unless you write some notes while you take the history. Remember, though, to try to make the patient your focus, rather than your notes, and be aware of the importance of eye contact to indicate that you are listening. One idea when you are learning to take histories is to sketch out the main headings beforehand and then write the history down in rough as you go along, filling in the bits of information as the patient offers them. You can then write it up neatly later. As you become more experienced, you will find that you will be able to dispense with the rough version of the note taking. In many hospitals, structured pro formas are increasingly being used to 'clerk' patients, and these are helpful to remember everything you need to cover (**Figure 4.1**).

Case notes (see **Figure 4.2**) are a treasure trove of information, and one of your key learning opportunities in clinical areas. Always read patients' notes when you get the opportunity, as in them you will find the clerking notes of other doctors, results of previous investigations the patient has had, and so on. Case notes look confusing at first, but as you get more experienced at understanding them, you will begin to piece together which symptoms indicate which diagnosis and how that condition was managed, and to see how the results of the investigations informed the diagnosis and management.

CLERKING PRO FORMA
HISTORY

NAME _____

DOB _____

AGE _____

SEX _____

OCCUPATION _____

ETHNICITY (relevant re thal, sickle etc.) _____

PRESENTING COMPLAINT

HISTORY PRESENTING COMPLAINT

PAST MEDICAL HISTORY (includes POH & PGH)

DRUGS   ALLERGIES

FAMILY HISTORY

SOCIAL HISTORY (includes smoking and alcohol)

SYSTEMS REVIEW
General

Cardiovascular system

Respiratory system

Gastrointestinal system

Genitourinary system

Fig. 4.1 Sample of patient clerking pro forma

```
                                              Age 94 years

 Consultations

 20.8.2008    Path. Lab.
              I: Urinary MC&S (*R99)

 29.8.2008    Path. Lab.
              I: Urinary MC&S (*R100)

 15.9.2008    Path. Lab.
              I: Urinary MC&S (*R101), Urinary MC&S (*R102)

 7.10.2008    Home visit
              O:chest clear HS v soft p 70 reg SR with a few
              ectopics; breathing is rather phlegmy; eating and
              drinking well; good Slovakian carer; discussed
              with Mrs ____ daughter; might be worth periodic
              urine tests; eg monthly for now; flu vaccine given
              T 36.3
```

Fig. 4.2 Example of case notes

The structure of the way the history is written is conventional and you should follow it, so that any other professional reading your notes will know where to look to find a specific piece of information:

Demographics

- The patient's name, gender, address, and date of birth

- Who referred them, if appropriate

- The name and address of their GP and next of kin, if not already recorded

- Who gave the history if not the patient (for example a parent)

- The date and time of the history and examination

History

- The presenting complaint(s)

- The history of the presenting complaint(s) – including medical (disease) and patient's (illness) perspective, including ideas, concerns, and expectations

- Past medical history

- Drug/allergy history

- Family medical history

- Personal and social history

- Systems review
  - General
  - Cardiovascular system
  - Respiratory system
  - Gastrointestinal system
  - Genitourinary system
  - Neurological system
  - Musculoskeletal system
  - Endocrine system

Physical examination

- General

- Skin

- Hands

- Locomotor system

- Respiratory system

- Cardiovascular system

- Breasts

- Lymph nodes

- Nervous system

- Abdomen

Differential diagnosis

Also known as the Impression and Problem List, this should include in list form the most likely possible diagnoses on the basis of the history and examination. Your hypotheses should include both the disease and the illness issues. Remember also that patients often have more than one thing wrong with them.

Plan of management

This would include any investigations required to confirm or rule out a possible diagnosis, and any treatment already given, for example immediate treatment given in the ambulance or in the accident and emergency department. You should include a working diagnosis, although if you are not sure then put a question mark after it, or write 'query', for example 'Query angina'. You should then list what treatment/management you propose for this patient.

Explanation and planning with patient

Finally, always record the substance of any discussions you have had with the patient and their family, what they have been told, and if appropriate any information given to gain consent – and if that consent has been forthcoming or withheld.

Abbreviations used in case notes

In an ideal world, abbreviations would never be used, as they risk ambiguity, particularly when in one branch of medicine an abbreviation might commonly mean one thing, whereas in another speciality, the same abbreviation might be widely used to signify something else. Different abbreviations may also be used in different countries. However, abbreviations *are* extensively used in case notes and you will have to come to terms with the most common ones, if only to be able to read the notes. When you present patients, you should not abbreviate.

ABBREVIATIONS USED IN CASE NOTES

Headings for the medical history

PC	presenting complaint
HPC	history of presenting complaint (sometimes H_xPC)
H_x	history
PMH	past medical history (sometimes PSH – past surgical history – is also used but usually PMH covers both)
PPH or PΨH	past psychiatric history
DH	drug history
SH	social history
FH	family history
SQ	systematic questions or SE – systems enquiry

Other abbreviations commonly used in the history

I_x	investigations
R_x	treatment
BO	bowels opened
PU	passing urine
SI	sexual intercourse
$K = {}^4/26\text{--}30$	menstrual cycle (meaning – period lasts for 4 days, coming on every 26–30 days)
G_3P_{2+1}	a woman who has been pregnant (gravid) three times, of which two

proceeded beyond the 28th week and one which ended before 28 weeks, either by termination or miscarriage – pronounced 'gravida three para two plus one'

$1/7$ $3/7$	1 day, 3 days, etc.
$1/12$ $8/12$	1 month, 8 months, etc.
@ $3/7$	at around 3 days, etc.

Abbreviations used in prescriptions

od	once daily
bd	twice daily
tds	three times a day
qds	four times a day
nocte	at night
mane	in the morning
prn	as required

Abbreviations used in the general examination

O/E or OE	on examination
E_x	examination
T	temperature
P	pulse
bpm	beats per minute
R	respiratory rate
rpm	respirations per minute
BP	blood pressure
mmHg	millimetres of mercury

SOB	short of breath or shortness of breath (or SOBOE – shortness of breath on exertion)		used in prescriptions to describe route of administration of drugs
NAD	no abnormalities detected	**NS**	**neurological system**
°	none or no, as in °palpitations = no palpitations, or °C = no cyanosis	CNS	central nervous system
		PERLA	pupils equal and reactive to light and accommodation
A	anaemia		
C	cyanosis	CN I–XII	1st to 12th cranial nerves
J	jaundice	P 3/5	power is grade 3 out of 5
club	clubbing	B, BR, KJ, AJ	biceps, brachioradialis, knee-jerk and ankle-jerk (reflexes)
lymph	lymphadenopathy		
HS	heart sounds	P↑ or P↓	plantar response up-going or down-going
TB	tuberculosis		
SR	sinus rhythm	**MS**	**musculoskeletal (system)** (or multiple sclerosis!)

Abbreviations used in the systems examinations

CVS	**cardiovascular system**
CVP	central venous pressure
PND	paroxysmal nocturnal dyspnoea
ECG	electrocardiograph
QRS	the wave form of an electrocardiograph
HS	heart sounds
JVP	jugular venous pressure (JVP↑ 15 cm = a jugular venous pressure raised by 15 cm)
PP	peripheral pulses
PSM	pan systolic murmur
5ICSMCL	fifth intercostal space, mid-clavicular line (i.e. where the atypical beat is normally felt)
RS	**respiratory system**
BS	breath sounds (in the context of respiratory examination, but can be bowel sounds in gastrointesinal system, or sometimes blood sugar!)
PN	percussion note(s)
AE	air entry
TVF	tactile vocal fremitus
exp	thoracic expansion on inspiration
creps	crepitus
GI or GIS	**gastrointestinal system**
LKKS	liver, kidneys, and spleen – °LKKS means no palpable liver, kidneys, or spleen
PR	per rectum – either rectal examination or rectal administration of drugs
PV	per vagina – again usually means examination, but can be

Other common medical abbreviations you might come across

AFB	acid-fast bacilli
AXR	abdominal X-ray
BCG	bacille Calmette–Guérin (vaccination against tuberculosis)
CT	computerized tomography
CXR	chest X-ray
EMU	early morning specimen of urine
ERCP	endoscopic retrograde cholangeopancreatogram
ESR	erythrocyte sedimentation rate
FBC	full blood count
Hb	haemoglobin
HbsAg	hepatitis B virus surface antigen
HC	head circumference
Hib	*Haemophilus influenzae*
ICP	intercranial pressure
IP	inpatient
LFT	liver function test
LVH	left ventricular hypertrophy
MCS	microscopy, culture, and sensitivities
MRI	magnetic resonance imagery
MSU	mid-stream specimen of urine
OP	outpatient
OT	occupational therapy
TAH	total abdominal hysterectomy
TOP	termination of pregnancy
U+Es	urea and electrolytes
US	ultrasound
WCC	white cell count

There are also conventional ways to document heart sounds, muscle strength, and level of consciousness, as well as ways to represent diagrammatically the presence or absence of palpable pulses, and the lungs and abdomen. You will find these conventions in any book on clinical skills; Cox & Roper (2005) is recommended.

Other forms of medical communication

Referral and discharge letters

Apart from the patients' records, one of the most common forms of written medical communication is letters written between healthcare professionals, for example referring a patient from a GP to a hospital, and vice versa when an inpatient is discharged.

Patients usually welcome the opportunity of having copies of their referral letters, and recently the practice of copying patients into their referral letters has become widespread. In the UK, The National Health Service Plan of 2000 directed that patients should be routinely offered copies of letters about themselves (Noble, 2007), as illustrated by **Figure 4.3**. Some doctors dislike the practice as it prevents them writing freely and frankly to other professionals (McConnell *et al.*, 1999), and some patients may not be able to understand the letters, particularly when medical terminology and jargon are used or when they have English as an

Dear Dr General Practitioner,

Re: Patient name, patient details

Diagnosis: Adenocarcinoma L breast 2005

Treatment: L wide local excision, tamoxifen

I saw Mrs _____ for her routine follow-up appointment on 12th Jan, and I am pleased to say that she is well, with no symptoms of recurrence. She continues to take tamoxifen. Physical examination was unremarkable except for a well-healed scar on the left breast. A mammogram performed on 11th Jan has been reported as normal. I have arranged to see her again in 6 months' time. In the meantime, please do not hesitate to contact us if you have any concerns.

Yours sincerely,

Mr Consultant Surgeon

Cc. Patient name

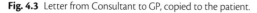

Fig. 4.3 Letter from Consultant to GP, copied to the patient.

Mr Consultant Surgeon
MBChB MD FRCS

Patient details

10 January 2007

Dear _____

I am pleased to tell you that your mammogram taken recently shows no signs of cancer. However, a very small number of breast cancers are not detected by screening and some can occur between screening, so it is important to be breast aware.

IF YOU NOTICE ANY CHANGE IN YOUR BREASTS YOU SHOULD CONTACT YOUR GP FOR FURTHER ADVICE.

Your next screening should be in about two years time.

Yours sincerely,

(signed by Mr Consultant Surgeon)

cc Dr General Practitioner
Enc.

Fig. 4.4 Sample medical correspondence, addressed to the patient and copied to the GP.

additional language. Abbreviations should be avoided in letters that patients will receive copies of. Another possibility is a separate explanation letter in patient-friendly language (**Figure 4.4**), or separate sections of the letter for patient and doctor (White, 2004). When writing letters to other doctors, the convention in the medical profession is that you do not criticize colleagues, even if, for example, another doctor has poorly managed the patient previously.

When you discharge a hospital inpatient or outpatient back into the care of their GP, you will need to write a discharge letter (**Figure 4.5**) outlining what has

happened to this person and what should happen next. A useful aide-mémoire for the content of a discharge letter is the acronym DOCTOR (North London Cancer Network, 2006), standing for:

Diagnosis and treatment

Options regarding treatment

Care plan and timescale to follow up

Told – what has the patient/family been told

Other agencies involved/referred to

Review – who, where, when

Print Date: 18 August 2008

GP Details

Patient details

Hospital No.
NHS No.
DOB
Date of Adm. 06/08/2008
Date of D/C 16/08/2008

Discharge Summary – Health Services for Elderly People

Consultant: DR _____ Department: HSEP Phone:

Problems/Diagnosis	**Actions**
Ulcerative Colitis	Under Dr _____ last seen in July 2008 – has had some history of wt loss and constipation therefore was reviewed by the gastro SpR on call who has advised for a CT Pneumocolon as an Outpatient
Hyponatraemia was initial reason for admission which was due to diuretics which have subsequently been stopped Underlying mild cognitive impairment Hypothyroidism	

Investigations:	CT Head – no SOL, INTRACRANIAL HAEMORRHAGE nA 115 ON ADMISSION AND 129 ON DISCHARGE. In view of some persisting hyponatraemia we have ordered urine osmolality and serum osmolality and are awaiting results. We would be grateful if you arrange for urine Na and urine & serum osmolality and further I_x of her mild hyponatraemia.
Function:	Mobile with Zimmer frame. Lives alone but has had section 2 and physio assessment for package of care to be inserted. Doubly continent. Independent with transfers. Forgetful at times.
Services:	Carers to visit od and OT to add some applications for home
Additional Comments:	A CT pneumocolon has been requested as an OP and we are trying to arrange for her to come in as an IP on a day case ward to have her bowel prep in view of her frailty and age.
Follow Up:	CT Pneumocolon as an OP
Place of Discharge:	Home with package of care
Allergies:	NKDA

					Pharmacy		
Drug name	**Dose**	**Route**	**Freq.**	**Duration**	**Clinical Check**	**Dispensing**	**Accuracy Check**
Ferrous sulphate	200mg	po	od	Continue	M	AD	

Fig. 4.5 Sample discharge letter

Audiotapes of consultations

As well as copying referral letters to patients, another way of providing reinforcing information is via the use of audiotapes of the consultation. This is sometimes done in cancer care settings, particularly in first 'bad news' consultations, to allow patients to listen again to the consultation when the initial shock and emotion have subsided. The advantages of this are that production of audiotapes is cheap and it does not encroach on clinical time to provide them. A review of eight randomized controlled trials from Australia, North America, and the UK found that people with cancer who received recordings or summaries found them useful to remind them of what was said, and to inform family members and friends about their illness and treatment, and most patients positively valued having a record of their consultation (Scott *et al.*, 2001). Another Australian study evaluated the provision of audiotapes of consultations with 52 cancer patients and found that almost all patients who elected to take home a tape listened to it, and most patients thought it was useful (Knox *et al.*, 2002).

Medical certificates

Another common form of written medical information that doctors are asked to provide is medical reports and certificates, an example of which can be seen in **Figure 4.6**. These are usually provided by the patient's GP, although a hospital doctor might need to provide a medical certificate for a hospital inpatient. Some medical reports and certificates are provided to confirm a patient's incapacity to work, and are necessary to claim welfare benefits, while others may be needed, for example, for insurance purposes or to gain certain employment. Sometimes doctors are asked to produce reports for adoption and fostering purposes, or for a patient to gain access to priority for social housing, and so on.

Usually such reports can be provided only by a doctor (not another health professional) and should follow an examination of the patient on the day, or the day before, the certificate is issued. When doctors receive a request for a medical certificate or report, the request should indicate clearly the information that is required, and only factual information that can be personally verified should be provided. All information about the patient is confidential, including the fact that they have been ill, and so the patient must consent to its release (British Medical Association, 2004).

Consent forms

Most of the time, a patient's consent is presumed, for example if they roll up their sleeves when you ask if you can take their blood pressure, then you can presume that they have consented to having it taken. Similarly, if you ask a patient if they agree to you examining them, and they verbally agree, then that is all that is required. However, when a medical intervention is complex, involves significant risks, or is part of a research programme, a written record of informed consent is needed (Noble, 2007). In such cases, only the doctor who will carry out the procedure should gain the patient's written consent. They will need to explain the risks and benefits of the procedure to the patient, and the record of the consent should contain some details about what was discussed, for example, whether there is likely to be postoperative pain, scarring, and any risk of long-term negative consequences. See Chapter 14 for further discussion of shared decision making and communicating risk.

The verbal discussion to 'inform' the written consent is probably the most important aspect from the patients' point of view, as research indicates that patients often do not read the consent form. For example, one UK study surveyed 256 patients who were undergoing surgery to test their recall of information and found that 69% of the patients admitted not reading the consent form before signing it, and those who did read it recalled no more information than those who did not (Lavelle-Jones *et al.*, 1993).

Summary

Good written communication is essential in ensuring continuity of patient care. It is also crucial when there are complaints, investigations, and litigation. The following is a useful summary of the content of good clinical records:

- History (relevant to the condition)
- Examination of the patient
- All systems examined
- All important findings, both positive and negative, with details of objective measurements such as blood pressure, peak flow, etc.
- Differential diagnosis
- Details of any investigations arranged
- Details of any referrals made
- Information given to the patient concerning risks and benefits of proposed treatment
- Details of patient consent to proposed investigations, treatments, or procedures

FOR SOCIAL SECURITY AND STATUTORY SICK PAY PURPOSES ONLY

NOTES TO PATIENT ABOUT USING THIS FORM

You can use this form either:

1. For Statutory Sick Pay (SSP) purposes – fill in Part A overleaf. Also fill in Part B if the doctor has given you a date to resume work. Give or send the completed form to your employer.
2. For Social Security purposes –
   To continue a claim for State benefit fill in Parts A and C of the form overleaf. Also fill in Part B if the doctor has given you a date to resume work. Sign and date the form and give or send it to your local Jobcentre Plus or Social Security office QUICKLY to avoid losing benefit.

NOTE: To start your claim to State benefit, if you are self-employed, or non-employed contact your Jobcentre Plus or Social Security office. If you are employed contact Your employer for a form SSP1.

Doctor's Statement

In confidence to
Mr/Mrs/Miss/Ms ---

I examined you today/yesterday and advised you that

(a) You need not   (b) You should refrain from work
    refrain from
    work   for*†--

                         OR until--

Diagnosis of your disorder
causing absence from work --

Doctor's remarks

Doctor's   Date of
signature   signing

Doctor's name and Health Authority   *Form Med 3*

NOTE TO DOCTOR*† *See inside front cover for notes on completion*

Fig. 4.6 Example medical certification

- Details of treatments, doses of drugs, and other treatments
- Arrangements for follow-up
- Progress, any further consultations, and how the patient has progressed (Medical Protection Society, 2008)

Further reading

In order to submit assignments for medical school, you will need to be able to write in an academic style. This aspect of written communication skills is outside the scope of this book, and if you feel you need extra help in this area, you should refer to a book such as:

Turner, K., Ireland, L., Krenus, B., and Pointon, L. (2007). *Essential Academic Skills.* Oxford: Oxford University Press.

Visit the Online Resource Centre for *Clinical Communication Skills* at: www.oxfordtextbooks.co.uk/orc/washer

References

British Medical Association (2004). *Medical Certificates and Reports.* London: British Medical Association.

Cox, L. and Roper, T. (2005). *Clinical Skills.* Oxford: Oxford University Press.

Department of Health (2002). *Building a Safer NHS for Patients: Implementing an Organisation with a Memory.* London: HMSO.

Knox, R., Butow, P.N., Devine, R., and Tattersall, M.H. (2002). Audiotapes of oncology consultations: Only for the first consultation? *Annals of Oncology*, **13**(4), 622–627.

Lavelle-Jones, C., Byrne, D.J., Rice, P., and Cuschieri, A. (1993). Factors affecting quality of informed consent. *British Medical Journal*, **306**(6882), 885–890.

McConnell, D., Butow, P.N., and Tattersall, M.H. (1999). Audiotapes and letters to patients: The practice and views of oncologists, surgeons and general practitioners. *British Journal of Cancer*, **79**(11/12), 1782–1788.

Medical Protection Society (2008). *MPS Guide to Medical Records.* London: Medical Protection Society.

Noble, L. (2007). Written communication. In: S. Ayers, A. Baum, C. McManus, S. Newman, K. Wallston, J. Weinman, and R. West (Eds), *Cambridge Handbook of Psychology, Health and Medicine.* Cambridge: Cambridge University Press, pp. 517–521.

North London Cancer Network (2006). *Communicating Significant News.* London: North London Cancer Care Network.

Scott, J.T., Entwistle, V.A., Sowden, A.J., and Watt, I. (2001). Giving tape recordings or written summaries of consultations to people with cancer: A systematic review. *Health Expectations*, **4**(3), 162–169.

White, P. (2004). Copying referral letters to patients: Prepare for change. *Patient Education and Counselling*, **54**(2), 159–161.

CHAPTER 5

Giving presentations

Katherine Woolf, Jayne Kavanagh, and Melissa Gardner

Learning points

This chapter will:

◆ outline some general presentation tips

◆ suggest ways to combat presentation anxiety

◆ provide specific tips for giving case presentations.

Presenting information orally is a key professional skill for medical students and doctors. Throughout your career, you will present information in a number of different contexts and situations, from the very formal (Grand Round presentations) to the informal (presentation to a friendly junior doctor). As you become more experienced, you will also begin to teach more junior students and, later, other doctors and healthcare professionals. However, giving oral presentations can be a terrifying experience for some; research shows that public speaking is often people's greatest fear (Cunningham *et al.*, 2006). This chapter will begin by describing some general presentation tips and will then provide you with some strategies for dealing with presentation anxiety. Finally, you will learn how to give a case presentation to your colleagues based on the medical history you learned how to take and write up in the previous two chapters.

General presentation tips

The following are some key general tips that you can use before, during, and after you give presentations in order to ensure you come across as slick and in control

– in short, as professional. It may seem as if there are lots of things to remember, but the more you practise, the easier it will become.

Preparing your presentation

The most important aspect of giving a presentation is making sure that your presentation is structured, with a clear introduction, body, and conclusion. It takes time and thought to provide your audience with information that is organized and logical. However, it is worth the effort because it makes it easier for you to understand and remember what you are telling them, and it makes you look and feel more in control of the information that you are presenting. It also makes it easier for your audience to understand and retain what you are telling them.

Just like when you present information in a written essay, all oral presentations should have an introduction, in which you set the scene, a body, in which you provide most of the information, and a conclusion, in which you summarize and signal the close of the presentation. When you are preparing your presentation, make sure it contains each of these elements.

Before you give your presentation, try to identify the main points you want to communicate to your audience. If your audience had to write down a few 'take home messages' they would learn from your presentation, what would you want those messages to be? Once you have identified what these key points are, try to put them in a logical order. There is generally no right or wrong way to do this, although sometimes there is a conventional way to organize information in certain types of presentation – this is discussed below. Once you have organized your key points, memorize the order in which they appear. This becomes the structure of the body of your presentation. If you know this off by heart, it is much harder to get lost while you are giving your presentation.

If you do get the opportunity to practise your presentation, it will help you feel more confident about delivering it, and will also help you to identify and correct any problems there may be with it. It is not always possible to practise a full presentation, so if you are short of time, try to practise just the opening lines – the beginning of a presentation is usually when you are most nervous, so practising these lines will help you feel more confident right from the start.

Answering questions from the audience is often perceived as one of the most daunting aspects of giving a presentation. One way to manage this is to try to think through in advance what questions you might possibly be asked and prepare answers to them before you give the presentation. By doing so, you will dramatically improve the answers you give, and also how you feel about answering any questions. In a case presentation, you are likely to be asked about differential diagnoses and possible investigations, so it is well worth preparing your answers to these questions beforehand. Particularly in clinical case presentations, it is important not to try to make up or guess the answers to difficult questions. It is safer and more professional to admit you do not know, and to say what you will do to find out.

During the presentation

A presentation is a form of communication, and building a rapport with your audience is an important part of the communicative process. Your audience will think you are a better presenter if you make them feel that they are an important part of the presentation, and one easy way to do this is to smile at them. Smiling also makes you look (and feel) relaxed and in control. Making eye contact is another basic way to build a rapport. It is also useful because it means you can respond to the way your audience is behaving. For example, if people are looking confused, you can slow down, check they have understood by asking them a question, or summarize the information you have given them. If people are smiling back at you, you can congratulate yourself!

Giving a presentation is a bit like being on stage: it is a performance. People will generally want to hear what you have got to say, and will want to understand it. This means you need to make sure you speak more loudly, clearly, and slowly than you would do normally. Projecting your voice is another tactic to make you seem more confident, in control, and relaxed.

Before the audience can take in the key information you are going to give them, they need some kind of lead in to get them in the right mode for listening. If they do not know you, this can be achieved by introducing yourself – telling them your name and some background information about yourself, including your experience in the subject you are going to be talking about. Having this information will help your audience trust you and trust what you are telling them. If your audience knows you and you feel you do not need to introduce yourself, the lead in could be a simple, brief sentence such as, **'I'm going to talk about a patient I've just seen'** or, **'We're going to be looking at . . .'** or, **'I was asked to read about (. . . this subject . . .) and tell you about it.'**

Early on in your presentation, you can tell your audience why they should listen to you: What's in it for them? What will they learn? What will they miss if they don't listen? Try using phrases like, **'This case was a particularly interesting case (or this is an important topic) because . . .'** For example, **'Twenty per cent of people in the UK have this condition, so it's important for all first-year clinical medical students to be able to recognize it.'**

One of the biggest advantages of presentations over other forms of learning is that there are opportunities for the audience and speaker to interact. Ideally, the interaction will be two-way, with you asking your audience questions, while also giving them the opportunity to ask you questions. This makes the audience feel involved, stops them becoming bored, and makes them feel you are interested in them and their ideas on the subject. In addition, interacting with the audience helps to build a rapport between you and the audience, and will encourage them to feel positive towards you. Interaction may not be appropriate in every situation, for example, it would not be appropriate for you to ask questions while you are presenting a patient to a senior consultant. However, when used appropriately, interacting with the audience can make the difference between a dull and an engaging presentation.

The conclusion of your presentation is your opportunity to summarize your key points. It is the final 'hammering home' of your message and should be the last thing your audience hears and remembers before they leave, or before you stop talking. Your summary can begin with the words, **'In summary, . . .'** and should be a very brief rundown of the key points of your presentation. It is very easy to forget to summarize, but this leaves your audience unsure about what to expect: Have you finished? Can they leave? Should they be doing something? It also leaves a rather unsatisfactory feeling in the air, whereas a solid conclusion leaves people feeling satisfied and gives them a sense of resolution. This will give the impression that you are a well-organized and professional person who knows what they are talking about.

After the presentation

Gaining insight into your performance is the best way of improving your subsequent presentations. Ask a person you trust to give you constructive feedback (see Chapter 6 in this book for a discussion about giving and receiving feedback). Try not to be too hard on yourself – giving presentations will become easier with practise and experience. In terms of case presentations, as a junior medical student with little clinical knowledge or experience, you may find it hard to think of differential diagnoses or possible investigations and management plans. Over time, you will become more experienced and knowledgeable, and these aspects will get easier.

How to deal with presentation anxiety

It is natural to suffer from some anxiety before giving a presentation, and adrenaline can often help you focus and perform well. Anxiety is most obvious to the person experiencing it, so although you may feel very anxious, your audience probably will not notice if your palms are sweating, your cheeks are flushed, your legs are wobbling, and your voice is shaking. Audience members have a lot of other things to think about: they may be preoccupied by the content of your presentation, how hot, cold, or tired they are, whether they have fed the cat, whether they have time to get a sandwich after your presentation, and so on. It is unlikely they will be concentrating on how nervous you appear.

If you do notice yourself starting to feel very nervous, concentrate on the audience. Try to judge whether they look interested in what you are saying. For example, are they nodding, looking away, or chatting? If they look confused, summarize the last few key points you have covered to help them understand. If they look cold, suggest somebody turns up the heating. If they look hot, suggest someone opens a window. Not only will this help your audience, but concentrating on them rather than yourself will shift your focus away from your own anxiety.

The following are some techniques you can use to minimize presentation anxiety. They probably will not remove your anxiety completely, but this is not a bad thing, as a certain degree of nervousness can help you perform effectively.

DEALING WITH PRESENTATION ANXIETY

- Prepare your presentation as far in advance as possible.
- Practise your presentation before you give it. (Give your opening and closing lines special attention – learn them by heart if you have time.)
- Remember that nerves are natural and can help you give a good performance.
- Remember that you feel much more nervous than you look.

◆ Remember that there is no such thing as a perfect presentation: it is okay to make some mistakes.

◆ During the presentation, concentrate on the audience rather than on how you are feeling.

◆ Make sure you get **constructive** feedback from someone you trust afterwards.

See Woolf & Kavanagh (2006) for a fuller account of dealing with presentation anxiety.

Giving case presentations

Giving a case presentation can be a daunting task. As a medical student, your clinical competence will be partly judged in both formative and summative assessments on your ability to give a good case presentation. The following are some tips for giving a case presentation on a ward round – although you can adapt them for giving case presentations in other settings. For example, see McGee & Irby (1997) for advice about giving case presentations in outpatients' clinics.

There are two key things to remember about case presentations: Firstly, there is no 'right' way to present a case. There are general principles for presenting cases, which will be discussed below, but in time you will find you develop your own particular presentation style. The second thing to remember is that the part of the presentation where you give the history of the presenting complaint is the key to the rest of the presentation.

The convention for giving information in a case presentation is analogous to the way case notes are written up (see Chapter 4) and is usually given in the following order:

◆ Presenting complaint (PC)

◆ History of the presenting complaint (HPC)

◆ Systems review

◆ Past medical history (PMH)

◆ Drug history (DH)

◆ Family history (FH)

◆ Social history (SH)

◆ Examination findings

◆ Case summary

◆ Differential diagnoses

◆ Planned investigations

◆ Initial management plans

Presenting complaint

Your opening sentence provides an overview of the presenting complaint and any other relevant background on the patient, for example their gender and age. The opening sentence should be short; you should be able to say it in one breath. Some examples of opening sentences, and the explanation for the information in each, are provided in Table 5.1.

History of the presenting complaint

The history of the presenting complaint is the longest and most complex part of the presentation. It details anything that might be relevant to the presenting complaint. A study of the ways in which doctors evaluate students' case presentations found that the score given to the history of the presenting complaint was strongly correlated with the overall score given to the

TABLE 5.1 Example opening sentences for case presentations, together with an explanation for the information included

Opening sentence	Explanation
'This man is a 35-year-old builder who was previously fit and well. He reports binge drinking and taking cocaine this weekend. He presented with chest pain…'	The patient's recent drinking and cocaine use is important because, in light of the fact that he was previously fit and well, it suggests that he might have drug-related cardiac pain.
'This young Somalian woman is a full-time English student. She is a known diabetic and is 22 weeks pregnant. She presented with shortness of breath…'	The fact that the patient is Somalian may be relevant to her shortness of breath. This may prompt you, and the listener, to think of and actively exclude certain diagnoses such as tuberculosis or HIV/AIDS.
'This woman is an 84-year-old nursing-home resident who requires care for all daily activities of living. She has a background of heart failure, COPD, and dementia. She presented with acute confusion…'	That the patient requires this much care and has a number of other medical complaints is relevant here because these facts will influence the treatment and the ways in which she will need to be cared for.

case presentation (Elliot & Hickam, 1997), so it is worth trying to make this part of your presentation as proficient as possible. Try to present the information in the order that it happened to the patient, even if the patient has not told you the information that way. For example, a patient who presents with shortness of breath may say that they felt particularly breathless the previous Tuesday and not mention until much later that the problem has been going on for 6 months. When you are presenting this information, it is useful to start by saying that the problem has been going on for 6 months and then lead on to the more recent events, as this structure makes the information clearer for the listener.

As well as stating the symptoms the patient has come with, you should state the presence or absence of any other symptoms that you think might be related to the presenting complaint. For example, if a patient presents with a cough, you should mention in the history of the presenting complaint whether a wheeze and shortness of breath is present or absent as well as mentioning whether they are producing sputum, their exercise tolerance, and so on. As your clinical experience and knowledge increases, this will become easier and you will start to recognize 'symptom sets': those types of symptoms that go together to suggest a particular diagnosis. Similarly, you will need to talk about the risk factors that are relevant to the presenting complaint, including any important risk factors that the patient *does not* have. This can be difficult without clinical experience, but there are some obvious risk factors you will be aware of and which you can mention – for example, risk factors for heart disease such as smoking, high cholesterol, and high blood pressure.

Systems review

You do not need to describe all the findings of your systems review in your case presentation, just mention the important, positive ones. For example, you should mention if a patient presents with a cough, but the systems review reveals they have changing bowel habits and blood in their stools. Despite the fact that the bowel findings are not related to the cough, some action will still need to be taken about them.

The rest of the history

The amount of detail you present will depend on your audience. For example, in an informal ward round you would only mention very significant diseases. However, when you are presenting a new patient to a consultant, you should provide more detail. When reporting the key aspects of the past medical history, it is important to try and give a time frame. For example, if a patient has diabetes, say when it was first diagnosed. When giving a drug history, you do not need to routinely mention doses or routes, but make sure you know these in case you are asked. Similarly, you should just mention positive findings and important negatives from a family history; for example, if a patient presents with chest pain, it is important to know that one of their parents died of a heart attack at age 50. You should begin the social history with the patient's occupation or any particular reasons why they are not currently working. Say who they live with and in what type of accommodation. Always talk about the patient's smoking and alcohol use, and mention recreational drugs if it seems appropriate.

Examination findings

Report the overall appearance of the patient on general inspection. For example, from the end of the bed, did they look jaundiced, obese, comatose? Say what you consider to be the key positive and negative findings from each system you examined. If you did not perform a particular examination and you think it might be relevant to the patient's problem (for example, the patient has abdominal pain and you did not perform a rectal examination), then you should state that it has not been performed.

Case summary

The summary of the case is similar to the opening sentence, but also includes the important positive and negative examination findings. Mention a few key points in the history such as important information about the pain, or a relevant medication that was recently started or stopped. Having a slick summary makes you look professional and knowledgeable. It is worth writing it out to ensure you have got it right and, again, practising it if you get the opportunity. It is also worth making a list of the patient's problems at this point, which you can then turn into a 'to do' list. This will help your team to think about how they might approach each problem on the list.

Differential diagnoses, investigations, and management plans

When you start giving case presentations and do not have much clinical experience, this part of the presentation may seem particularly difficult. However, suggesting differential diagnoses shows that you are thinking about the clinical problem already. Naturally, as you get more experienced, you will be able to provide a fuller and more confident account of the possible diagnoses, any investigations that might need to be ordered, and what should be done for this patient. It is generally better to mention less invasive, simpler procedures before you mention more complex ones. If your patient has complex problems, it might help to refer back to the problem list to know which investigations you want to order. It may be the case that investigations have already been ordered or completed, or that some treatments have already been initiated. In this case, you may want to do the case summary of your presentation at this point, rather than earlier, so as to include this information.

If a patient has been in hospital for some time, you do not need to pretend that the patient has just been admitted. Instead, say when they came into hospital in the opening sentence of your presentation. Summarize the presenting complaint, history of the presenting complaint, drug history, family history, social history, and examination findings as they were at the time of admission, but instead of giving the case summary, present the patient's progress in hospital and say how the patient is currently. A patient who has been in hospital for a while will probably have received a diagnosis, so it does not make sense to state your differential diagnoses at this point. However, you might be asked what differential diagnoses you would have considered if you had seen the patient when they were first admitted, so it is worth thinking about this before you present.

Summary

Giving presentations is a key skill required of all professionals, and in medicine it is an important way of learning and being assessed. By preparing your presentations using the good practice guidelines outlined in this chapter, you will ensure that they are professional and engaging. Everyone experiences some degree of anxiety about giving presentations, but try to use that anxiety to help focus your presentation skills rather than let your anxiety get in the way of what you want to say.

Further reading

Woolf, K. and Kavanagh, J. (2006). Giving presentations without palpitations. *British Medical Journal Careers Focus*, **332**, 242–243.

Visit the Online Resource Centre for *Clinical Communication Skills* at: www.oxfordtextbooks.co.uk/orc/washer

References

Cunningham, V., Lefkoe, M., and Sechrest, L. (2006). Eliminating fears: An intervention that permanently eliminates the fear of public speaking. *Clinical Psychology and Psychotherapy*, **13**(3), 183–193.

Elliot, D. and Hickam, D. (1997). How do faculty evaluate students' case presentations? *Teaching and Learning in Medicine*, **9**(4), 261–263.

McGee, S. and Irby, D. (1997). Teaching in the outpatient clinic: Practical tips. *Journal of General Internal Medicine*, **12**(S2), S34–S40.

Woolf, K. and Kavanagh, J. (2006). Giving presentations without palpitations. *British Medical Journal Careers Focus*, **332**, 242–243.

CHAPTER 6

Talking with other health professionals and patients' families

Peter Washer

Learning points

This chapter will:

♦ discuss the importance of multidisciplinary team working

♦ discuss how to use the multidisciplinary team as a learning resource

♦ describe best practice in giving and receiving feedback

♦ discuss the issues that arise when talking with patients' families.

Clinical communication is often conceived as being only about doctors talking with their patients. However, just as important is communication with other doctors, with other healthcare professionals, with other professionals such as social workers, managers and lawyers, and with patients' families. One major trend in healthcare generally is an increasing flexibility in the workforce: the breaking down of previous occupational barriers and the opening up of new opportunities for the development of skills to fill perceived shortages. For example, the number and diversity of specialist nurse practitioners, GPs with 'a special interest' in specific types of patient, and new occupations such as non-medically qualified 'surgical care practitioners' have increased to undertake tasks that previously were the sole reserve of doctors (Sanders & Harrison, 2008). These developments again underline the need for effective team working.

This chapter will describe how, as a student, you can use the diversity of the multidisciplinary team (MDT) as a learning resource and will discuss the importance of MDT working and safe handovers of patient care. Giving and receiving feedback among colleagues is a key part of medical education, and this chapter will give some best practice advice in that area. The final part of this chapter looks at the issues that can arise when talking to patients' families, and will describe best practice when using the telephone to talk to patients and their families.

Learning from the multidisciplinary team

Clinical areas are packed full of learning opportunities, but those opportunities will not come and find you if you don't put yourself 'out there'. When you first go into a new clinical area, introduce yourself to the various people who work there, chat to them, and ask them about their work. As long as you are polite and friendly without being pushy, they will more often than not be happy to talk to you if they are not too busy. You will gain extra 'brownie points' if you can make yourself useful – offer to run errands and make people coffee. Be up front about your naivety, and charm people by acknowledging that they are much more experienced than you are, and you want them to share their expertise with you.

Often, an efficient receptionist or practice manager will be the best person to befriend when you need to track down case notes, or ask who is being admitted or discharged that day. Someone doing the hands-on care, such as a student nurse or healthcare assistant, is usually the best person to ask about whether a patient has managed to eat breakfast or has slept well. The Registered Nurses (Staff Nurses) will be allocated to looking after particular patients, and they are the people to ask whether patients are well enough or will be suitable for you to talk to. Ward managers (Sisters) will know when there are patients with interesting or unusual conditions on the ward. Ask the physiotherapists, occupational therapists, and speech and language therapists about their work. Pharmacists are a treasure trove of information about medicines. If a patient is going for an unusual investigation, ask if you can go with them to see it, and when you get to the department where the investigation is going to take place, ask the radiographer or doctor there to explain it to you.

The more senior people become in any profession, the busier they generally are. The consultant on your team may be a Head of Department, a professor and a world expert in their field, but you are going to have to compete for their time if you want them to teach you. More junior doctors are generally more approachable, and are closer to the student phase of their careers, so they will be able to identify with your level of knowledge and experience. As such, they are often good teachers. Remember that every member of the MDT is a busy professional with a job to do, so always ask them nicely when would be best for them to spare you their time, and of course always say please and thank you.

Working as part of a multidisciplinary team

As a doctor, you will be working as part of a team, and good communication between members of that team is essential for several reasons:

- Firstly, because patients have contact with many members of the team, and from their perspective a coordinated approach is reassuring.

PODCAST

A patient's perspective

"Why did you trust them [the multidisciplinary breast care team] and take the [treatment] option that they were favouring? What was it about them?"

"... The consultant himself was very knowledgeable, didn't patronize me, pitched the information at a level that I felt was appropriate, and there was a very, very integrated approach of the breast care nurses, and from the start there was a dedicated breast care unit there. I felt that the consultants and all the associated staff worked very well together as a team and I felt that in my particular case, the consultant had mentioned that he'd looked at the information in my patient records and had plotted sort of statistics and this was the option they were recommending, and I felt that my specific circumstances had been put in the context of wider population studies."

Podcast – Roisin, patient with breast cancer

- Secondly, poor communication within the team has been identified as an underlying factor in failed communication with patients, for example when conflicting information is given to patients by different members of the team (BMA Board of Medical Education, 2004). For example, one UK study surveyed five MDT breast cancer care teams, and found that there were many professionals involved in major discussions with the patient without the rest of the team's knowledge, with the risk of providing contradictory information to patients (Jenkins *et al.*, 2001).

◆ Thirdly, effective communication with other members of the MDT is important because research shows that doctors feel considerably less stressed when they feel they are part of a good team. For example, a Canadian study of 182 doctors found that the support the team members offered one another shielded them from the negative effects of work demands and was directly related to doctor well-being (Wallace & Lemaire, 2007). Similarly, research suggests that other health professionals find MDT working a source of satisfaction and motivation, although participation tends to follow traditional professional/occupational hierarchies, with nurses more likely to be 'talked over' by doctors (Lanceley *et al.*, 2008).

Handovers

When junior doctors worked long hours, individual continuity of care was possible. However, within the European Union at least, the working week is now limited to 48 hours, which effectively limits doctors to spending a maximum of 13 hours in the hospital each day. Whereas nurses have always worked shift patterns, now shift working has also become the norm for many doctors, at least in hospitals. The implication of changing to a shift pattern of working is that different teams will be looking after the same group of patients over the course of any given day, which in turn means that there have to be systems for effective handovers between shifts to protect patient safety (British Medical Association, 2004). Best practice in handovers is outlined in the box.

Talking with the media

Sometimes a patient in your care is newsworthy, for example you might have a patient who is a celebrity, or you might have patients injured following a disaster such as a bombing or train crash, or suffering from an unusual disease, such as SARS for example. In these types of circumstance, journalists will often try to find out information about them without using the proper channels, so you should be extremely careful about

---

BEST PRACTICE IN HANDOVERS

◆ The key handover to or from the night team should be multidisciplinary, and involvement of senior clinicians is essential.

◆ Handover should be at a fixed time and of sufficient length.

◆ This period should be known to all staff and designated 'bleep-free', except for immediately life-threatening emergencies.

◆ Shifts for all staff involved should be coordinated to allow them to attend in working time, particularly for the handover to and from the night team.

◆ Handovers will also be needed in the morning and at the change of other shifts (for example 5 p.m. in some ward settings).

◆ Handover should be supervised by the most senior clinician present.

◆ Information presented should be succinct and relevant, ideally, supported by information systems identifying all relevant patients.

Written (or IT-based) handover should include:

◆ current inpatients

◆ accepted and referred patients due to be assessed

◆ accurate location of all patients – use of bed/bay numbers should be avoided to prevent misidentification

◆ operational matters directly relevant to clinical care such as intensive care bed availability

◆ information to convey to the following shift

◆ patients whose condition is of particular concern.

As well as the above, a verbal handover should be given of:

◆ patients with anticipated problems, to clarify management plans and ensure appropriate review

◆ outstanding tasks, associated with their required time for completion.

British Medical Association (2004)

---

any confidential patient data you might inadvertently release. For example, if you are working in an AIDS care setting and someone phones and asks to speak to a patient, just by saying, '**I'll check to see if they want to** speak to you . . .' in effect confirms both that that person is there and their diagnosis. Instead, always take the caller's name and say, **'I'll just check if we have anyone on the ward of that name'**, and then check with the patient whether they know the caller and want to speak to them. If in doubt, err on the side of caution. Each hospital will have specialist press officers who will advise you on communicating with the media, and any dealings with the press are best left to them, unless you are trained and specifically given clearance by them to do otherwise.

Giving and receiving feedback

As a medical student and doctor, you need to learn to receive and process feedback. You will also often be asked to give feedback to fellow students, to your teachers in the form of course evaluations, and to other doctors. For example, in the UK, trainee doctors are now involved in a multisource feedback, with assessment from eight raters, both medical and non-medical, an approach that is relevant to assessing performance in a multidisciplinary workplace (Carr, 2006).

Getting feedback on how well you are progressing is an essential part of the educational process. Students sometimes neglect formative feedback as if it did not matter, because it does not count towards your final marks. However, formative feedback is arguably more important than summative (final) assessment, because it gives you an opportunity to work with the feedback to build on your strengths and address any weaknesses *before* you are assessed summatively.

Giving feedback on communication skills performance is often done in a formulaic way. This is sometimes called 'Pendleton's rules' after Pendleton *et al.* (1984):

- After a student has done a role play, they are invited to comment on what went well.

- Then the rest of the group is asked to suggest anything else that went well.

- The facilitator (and the simulated patient) then highlight what they thought went well.

- Then the student is asked to suggest anything that they would do differently in future.

- Again the group is asked to add to this, often suggesting alternative ways that things could have been done.

- Finally, the positive elements are reiterated.

GUIDELINES FOR GIVING FEEDBACK

Feedback should:

- be given sensitively, with both the giver and receiver working together, with common goals

- be asked for and expected, and given as close to the event as possible; it should not take the person receiving it by surprise

- be given by someone who has observed the person's performance first-hand, and selectively address one or two key issues rather than too many at once

- be limited to behaviours that can be changed, rather than to personality

- describe behaviour in concrete terms, for example, **'The differential diagnosis didn't include the possibility of . . .'**, rather than **'Your differential diagnosis was inadequate.'** Use tentative words such as **'sometimes'** and **'perhaps'**, rather than words like **'always'** and **'never'**, but do not be too apologetic, as this can imply that you feel that the person cannot handle what you are saying.

- deal with specific performances, not generalizations, for example **'Your time management is awful!'**

- be subjective, for example, **'When you were talking about the patient's cancer, I noticed you looked uncomfortable'**, rather than, **'You looked uncomfortable talking about the patient's cancer.'** Better still, just describe what you saw: **'I saw your hands were shaking and you changed the subject.'**

- deal with decisions and actions, rather than assumed intentions or interpretations, for example, **'The antibiotic wouldn't have provided coverage for . . .'** rather than, **'Your choice of antibiotic shows you didn't think about the possibility of . . . infection.'** Explain any consequences of their actions

- separate feedback from judgements by describing your emotional response: For example, rather than saying, **'That was disrespectful of you'**, you might say **'You used a term which many people might find offensive'** or, **'I don't think that's a good word to use because . . .'** (Burack *et al.*, 1999).

From Ende (1983)

Students tend to be very hard on their own performance, and one of the advantages of following this formula is that it moves the focus away from self-criticism at the outset and ensures that praise is given for what was good, so strengths can be built on. However, the rigid structure of Pendleton's rules has also been criticized, as it can become predictable and can inhibit spontaneous discussion of points as they occur. It is also difficult to avoid the perception that the feedback is contrasting 'good points' with 'bad points' despite the careful use of language (Carr, 2006).

Sometimes people react badly to feedback, becoming defensive and hostile. This possibility will be minimized if the giving of feedback is handled sensitively, using the guidelines above. King (1999) offers some strategies for dealing with bad reactions if they happen:

◆ Name and explore the resistance: **'You seem bothered by this – can you tell me why?'**

◆ Keep the focus positive: **'Let's recap your strengths and see if we can build on any of these to address the problem.'**

◆ Try to convince the person to own part of the problem: **'So would you accept that on that occasion you lost your temper?'**

◆ Negotiate: **'I can help with this, but first you need to . . .'**

◆ Allow time out: **'Do you need some time to think about this?'**

◆ Explore the resistance to understand it: **'Help me understand more about why you seem so angry.'**

◆ Keep the responsibility where it belongs: **'What will you do to address this?'**

Talking with patients' families

Families sometime ask doctors to breach confidentiality and provide information to them without the patient's knowledge or consent, or to withhold information from the patient, feeling that 'they wouldn't be able to cope'. As described in Chapter 8, there may also be cultural influences on family expectations. For example, a Japanese study of 74 hospital doctors found that, while in Western countries respect for individual autonomy is central, in Japan the best interests of both patients and families are taken into consideration. Japanese doctors would not therefore be expected to inform a patient of a fatal illness without the consent of the family (Akabayashi *et al.*, 1999).

Commonly, family members will ask students to give them information about the patient's condition, either because they feel the student is more approachable or because they have already tried to ask the qualified staff and have not got the information they wanted from them. If this happens, remind them that you are a medical student and tell them you will ask a doctor or a nurse to come and talk to them. There is detailed advice on giving information without providing false reassurance in Chapter 12 of this book.

When you *are* a doctor, discussing a patient's care with relatives can be difficult. Research indicates that patients want their autonomy to be respected when doctors talk to their families, and want to be told the truth themselves and have their confidentiality respected in discussions between their doctors and their families. For example, a UK study of 30 cancer patients found that they all wanted their doctors to respect their views rather than those of their family, should they differ. All also wanted their close family to receive information, but only with their consent, and they did not feel that without their consent, their families had a 'right' to information about them. Almost all were opposed to the idea of their family influencing the information that they themselves would receive about their own illness (Benson & Britten, 1996). In general, the patient should be given the information, and they can then pass on whatever information they want to their family. If a patient is conscious, you should always ask them whether they are happy for you to talk to their relatives. If a patient is unconscious or lacks capacity, you will need to make a professional judgement about how much you should tell the relatives, based on what is in the patient's best interests, taking into consideration their wishes if they are known. Doctors, especially junior doctors, should seek advice if uncertain (Medical Protection Society, 2008).

Although patients themselves must have the final say on information given to their families, at the same time it is important to acknowledge that families need support. Taking into account the advice above, families should be kept updated and have opportunities for any concerns they have to be addressed. Ideally, they should have the contact details of a key named professional involved in the patient's care – either a doctor or a nurse – to whom they can direct their questions. As discussed in Chapter 4, any discussions with relatives should be recorded in the patient's notes, so that other professionals are clear about what has been said to them.

A relative's perspective

"... within a couple of weeks we went into two different hospitals. The first hospital was extremely busy. We didn't really have any explanation of what was happening or what they were doing and we spent quite a number of hours there, really without proper information as to what they were doing. Basically I still didn't know what was wrong with him.

The second hospital we went to was very different in that they were less rushed. Perhaps it was a less busy time or perhaps a less busy hospital altogether in the A&E, but it was less rushed and whether it was a nurse or a doctor, somebody came every hour or half hour to tell us what they were going to do next, which was all we needed. Then you feel more at ease and less pressured."

"So it sounds like the issue is not that you were kept waiting – because you were obviously prepared for that – but that you were kept waiting without being given explanations of what was going on, and that was what was really important for you."

"Yes, exactly. Waiting in A&E or at any time in hospital is something we expect in a sense, but waiting without being told what's going to happen makes it far more stressful. We are already under pressure certainly if someone has been taken suddenly to hospital and they're very ill. Then we're already under a great deal of pressure and stress, and therefore we need to have feedback and to be put at ease that things are going to be done."

Podcast – Alice, carer for her partner

Using the telephone to talk with patients and relatives

Doctors use the telephone in a number of contexts, so it is worth considering best practice when using the telephone. Most of the following applies to talking on the phone with patients, their relatives, and other professionals. Using the phone can help patients and relatives by saving time and travel costs, particularly for people who might have to arrange child care or lose work time (Toon, 2002). Using telephone reminders reduces missed appointments, and can increase uptake of vaccinations and aid health promotion. After discharge, telephone contact with patients can provide opportunity for feedback on the care provided, inform patients of investigations, and check they understand any advice given. Providing telephone-based care does also carry a potential risk of missing a serious condition (Car & Sheikh, 2003); however, in certain contexts it can improve health outcomes. For example, research on the efficacy of using the telephone to review asthma patients rather than face-to-face consultations has shown that telephone reviews did not compromise either the patient's health or their satisfaction, were more efficient in terms of time, and more patients were reviewed (Pinnock *et al.*, 2003).

A SUGGESTED APPROACH TO A TELEPHONE CONSULTATION:

- Answer the telephone promptly.
- State your name.
- Obtain the caller's name and telephone number (in case the patient has to be called back by another member of the team or the call is disconnected).
- Speak directly with the person who has the problem.
- Record the date and time of the call.
- Record the person's details.
- Take an appropriately detailed and structured history and record it as you would in a face-to-face consultation.
- Provide advice on treatment and again record what advice has been given.
- Advise about follow-up and when to contact a doctor (for example, if symptoms are worsening or fail to improve despite treatment, or if there are new symptoms).
- Summarize the main points covered.
- Request the caller to repeat the advice given.
- Ask if the person has any outstanding questions or concerns.
- Let the caller disconnect first.

From Car & Sheikh (2003)

Finally, it is sometimes necessary to telephone relatives from hospital when a patient has died. It is not uncommon for junior doctors to have to do this, especially if the death happens at night. In the past, it was common practice for relatives to be phoned and told that the patient had deteriorated and for news of the death to be broken when they arrived at the hospital. However, this often led to relatives becoming angry and mistrustful if they later found out that the person had already died when they were called.

IF YOU HAVE TO PHONE RELATIVES TO INFORM THEM THE PATIENT HAS DIED:

- Make sure you check to whom you are speaking.

- Introduce yourself carefully, and say if you have already met them or another member of their family.

- Speak slowly and clearly, and give them time to adjust, particularly if it is the middle of the night.

- Fire a warning shot – for example, tell them you have some bad news about their relative and you would prefer to be able to tell them in person.

- Tell them, **'I'm sorry, but [the patient] has died.'** Use the word 'died', rather than 'passed away', 'passed over', 'we've lost them', and so on, which in the heat of the moment can be unclear.

- Ask who is with them, and suggest they get someone to support them if possible.

- Give them your contact details or the contact details of someone else on your team who is involved in the patient's care.

- Suggest they make contact with their GP and make sure the GP is informed of the death.

- If they are coming to the hospital, speak to them about how they can make the journey safely (is there someone who can drive them?) and make sure someone is there to greet them when they arrive and to take them to the deceased.

- If they are not coming to the hospital, make sure they understand the practicalities of the next stage, and how to contact any bereavement services available.

Adapted from North London Cancer Network (2006)

Summary

Medical students need to learn to talk not just with patients, but with a whole range of people. As a doctor, you will need to communicate effectively with a range of experts and lay people. Remember that other professionals have expertise that you do not have, and use them as a resource to learn from. When talking with relatives, check where possible that the patient has agreed what their family should be told. Colluding with relatives to keep information from patients is bad practice and should be avoided.

Further reading

Visit the Online Resource Centre for *Clinical Communication Skills* at: www.oxfordtextbooks.co.uk/orc/washer

References

Akabayashi, A., Kai, I., Takemura, H., and Okazaki, H. (1999). Truth telling in the case of a pessimistic diagnosis in Japan. *The Lancet*, **354**(9186), 1263.

Benson, J. and Britten, N. (1996). Respecting the autonomy of cancer patients when talking with their families: Qualitative analysis of semi-structured interviews with patients. *British Medical Journal*, **313**(7059), 729–731.

BMA Board of Medical Education (2004). *Communication Skills Education for Doctors: An Update*. London: British Medical Association.

British Medical Association (2004). *Safe Handover, Safe Patients. Guidance on Clinical Handover for Clinicians and Managers*. London: British Medical Association.

Burack, J.H., Irby, D.M., Carline, J.D., Root, R.K., and Larson, E.B. (1999). Teaching compassion and respect: Attending physicians' responses to problematic behaviors. *Journal of General Internal Medicine*, **14**(1), 49–55.

Car, J. and Sheikh, A. (2003). Telephone consultations. *British Medical Journal*, **326**(7396), 966–969.

Carr, S. (2006). The Foundation Programme assessment tools: An opportunity to enhance feedback to trainees? *Postgraduate Medical Journal*, **82**(576), 579.

Ende, J. (1983). Feedback in clinical medical education. *Journal of the American Medical Association*, **250**(6), 777–781.

Jenkins, V., Fallowfield, L., and Poole, K. (2001). Are members of multidisciplinary teams in breast cancer aware of each other's informational roles? *Quality in Health Care*, **10**(2), 70–75.

King, J. (1999). Giving feedback. *British Medical Journal*, **318**(7200), S2.

Lanceley, A., Savage, J., Menon, U., and Jacobs, I. (2008). Influences on multidisciplinary team decision-making. *International Journal of Gynaecological Cancer*, **18**, 215–222.

Medical Protection Society (2008). *MPS Guide to Medical Records*. London: Medical Protection Society.

North London Cancer Network (2006). *Communicating Significant News*. London: North London Cancer Care Network.

Pendleton, D., Schofield, T., Tate, P., and Havelock, P. (1984). *The Consultation: An Approach to Learning and Teaching*. Oxford: Oxford University Press.

Pinnock, H., Bawden, R., Proctor, S., Wolfe, S., Scullion, J., Price, D., and Sheikh, A. (2003). Accessibility, acceptability, and effectiveness in primary care of routine telephone review of asthma: Pragmatic, randomised controlled trial. *British Medical Journal*, **326**(7387), 477–479.

Sanders, T. and Harrison, S. (2008). Professional legitimacy claims in the multidisciplinary workplace: The case of heart failure care. *Sociology of Health and Illness*, **30**(2), 289–308.

Toon, P.D. (2002). Using telephones in primary care. *British Medical Journal*, **324**(7348), 1230–1231.

Wallace, J. and Lemaire, J. (2007). On physician well being – You'll get by with a little help from your friends. *Social Science & Medicine*, **64**, 2565–2577.

CHAPTER 7

Talking with disabled people

Peter Washer

Learning points

This chapter will:

- discuss the changes in social attitudes to disability
- describe some strategies to help you talk with people with speech and language impairments
- describe ways to communicate with people with different sensory impairments
- examine the communication issues for people with profound learning disabilities and ways of assessing their needs.

One of the more positive social changes over the past generation or so has been a fundamental rethink about the way that society treats disabled people. Since the 1970s, disabled people around the world have argued that changes in the law are needed to protect them from discrimination, just as there have been changes in the law in many countries to protect people from discrimination on racial and religious grounds. In many countries, this lobbying has resulted in legislation prohibiting discrimination against disabled people, for example, in the USA (The Americans with Disabilities Act 1990), in Australia (The Disability Discrimination Act 1992), and in the UK (The Disability Discrimination Act 1995 and 2005), as well as elsewhere. European Human Rights legislation has also been fundamental. This type of legislation generally places a duty on all public bodies such as healthcare providers and educational institutions to provide equal access to services and opportunities for disabled people so that they can participate in work and public life. The aim of this legislation is to actively promote disability equality and positive attitudes and to tackle 'disablism' – discriminatory, oppressive, or abusive behaviour arising from the belief that disabled people are inferior to others (Miller *et al.*, 2004).

Although there is a tendency for most of the general public to think of disabled people as wheelchair users, only about 4% of disabled people use a wheelchair. During a career in medicine, you will encounter many people with different types of disabilities, some of which will affect their ability to communicate more than others. Before looking at the specific communication needs relating to some types of disability, it will be useful to give some background to the changes in language and attitudes to contextualize the communication issues.

Different models of disability

The medical model of disability sees the doctor's role as either to *cure* the *patient*, or else to help *carers manage* the *problem* so that the patient can *fit in* to society and live as *normal* a life as possible. The social model of disability, by contrast, regards society's reaction to disabled people, rather than their impairments, as what makes their lives so unnecessarily difficult. Disabled people have argued for a move away from the medical model and to the social model of disability. The opposite of disabled is not able-bodied or abled, but non-disabled or *enabled*.

The language used by both doctors and lay people to describe disabled people only a generation ago seems shockingly insensitive now. Words like cripple, spastic, cretin, idiot, mongol, retarded, and handicapped (derived from the times when disabled people begged on the streets 'cap in hand'), which were all once neutral medical terms, have become tainted with prejudice and have rightly been abandoned as pejorative. Those words have been replaced with words chosen by disabled people to describe themselves. Every disabled person will have their own views on what language they want to be used to describe them. The important thing if you are not sure about what words to use is to ask the person – and be prepared to be corrected.

Some of the impairments that lead to disability will not cause any particular communication difficulties. For the purposes of the rest of this chapter, we might want to distinguish between those impairments that cause problems relating to mobility, and those that cause difficulties with speech or language, or are sensory or intellectual. The remained of this chapter will therefore focus on those impairments that can raise particular communication issues, namely speech, hearing, sight, and severe learning impairments. The conclusion of this chapter will revisit the role of the doctor in dealing with disability more generally.

Talking with people with disorders of speech and language

As a medical student or junior doctor, you will most commonly encounter people with speech and language problems as a result of common conditions of older people such as Parkinson's disease or cerebrovascular accident (CVA or stroke). However, younger people can also develop speech and language impairments, for example following a head injury, or as a result of neurological conditions such as brain tumours and infections. Conditions such as multiple sclerosis or motor neurone disease can lead to a gradual slurring of speech, called dysarthria. People who have cancer of the larynx may have to have a laryngectomy – the surgical removal of their larynx. As a result, they totally lose their voice. Remember that some people (with cerebral palsy, for example) may be unable to control and coordinate the muscles required for speaking, but they may not have any learning disability.

A sudden loss of language can be particularly shattering and terrifying, especially where people are unable to understand explanations and cannot ask questions. People often have to mourn the loss of their previous self and learn new ways to communicate, such as gesture, communication boards, and mechanical devices. Our voice is so much a part of our identity that without it we can be left feeling diminished, humiliated, socially isolated, and depressed (Dalton, 1994).

Dysphasia (sometimes called aphasia) is an umbrella term for problems with understanding and expressing spoken and written language. Dysphasia is associated with common conditions such as stroke, brain tumour, and head injuries. People with dysphasia may have little or no comprehension or they may be able to process only simple language. Although dysphasia does not affect reasoning ability, people may have problems with finding words, structuring sentences, and following a train of thought aloud.

Strategies for communicating with people with dysphasia

The National Institute on Deafness and Other Communication Disorders (1997) suggests these strategies for communicating with people with dysphasia:

- Try to find out from the patient and those close to them what strategies they use to communicate.

- Expect to take longer to communicate with them and don't try to hurry.

- Speak slowly but do not distort your speech.

- Use plain English and no jargon (as you should with all patients).

- Cover one topic at a time.

- Speak in short, simple sentences, without long clauses or deviations.

- Use closed and checking questions to clarify that you have understood each other.

- Be aware of the importance of non-verbal communication on both sides, especially gesture, pointing, and eye contact.

- Use diagrams, drawings, and writing, and if the patient is able to, encourage them to do the same.

Talking with people with sensory impairments

People who are deaf or hard of hearing

The term 'deaf' is a general term used to describe people anywhere on a broad spectrum of hearing loss. The word 'Deaf' written with a capital 'D' usually refers to people who consider themselves to be part of the Deaf community, which sees itself as a cultural or linguistic minority. The Deaf community does not consider deafness an impairment, and may therefore be unhappy with the term 'hearing impairment'. 'Hard of hearing' describes a person who has some level of hearing loss, which they may have had since childhood or acquired later. 'Partially deaf' or 'partially hearing' describes someone with some degree of hearing loss, either moderate or severe. Other terms such as 'deaf and dumb' or 'deaf mute' are now considered unacceptable and offensive (Hearing Concern, 2006a).

People who are deaf may use a range of strategies to communicate. The Deaf community use Sign Language as their first or preferred language. Sign Language has its own grammar and there are different regional versions, so although North American and British spoken English are mutually intelligible, American Sign Language and British Sign Language are not. Like any language, Sign Language takes time to learn, so a qualified Sign Language interpreter may be necessary to communicate effectively with a Deaf person. (See Chapter 8 for further information on how to work with interpreters.) Most hard of hearing people communicate using speech, possibly combined with a hearing aid and lip-reading. One rule of thumb when you meet a person who you know to be deaf or hard of hearing is always to explore with them which way they prefer to communicate. Also, if they do use a hearing aid, check that it is on and if it is working.

TIPS TO HELP YOU COMMUNICATE IF A PERSON IS DEAF OR HARD OF HEARING

The following range of advice has been produced from a number of sources (Byron *et al.*, 2006; Hearing Concern, 2006b; RNID, 2006; Sense, 2003, 2006)

The environment

- Reduce or minimize any background noise.

- Ensure that the room and your face are well lit and that any direct light is on your face (and behind the person).

- Avoid bright sunlight or lights that can dazzle and make lip-reading impossible.

- Check how close and in what position you need to be so that the person can hear and see you as clearly as possible – usually standing 3–6 feet apart if the person is lip-reading. You may need to move closer or to one side if the hearing is better in one ear.

Introduce yourself

- Make sure that you have the person's attention before speaking. A light touch on the arm, a wave, or another visual signal will help when you introduce yourself.

- Check with the person whether the level and pace of your speech is right for them.

- The context is important in aiding understanding, so give the subject of the conversation first and warn the person if you are changing the subject.

While speaking

- Look directly at the person when speaking (even if an interpreter is present).

- Maintain eye contact and keep your head fairly still.

- Keep your hands away from your face and mouth.

- Speak normally and clearly with a normal speech rhythm, but if you do usually talk quickly, slow down slightly.

- Try to make your lip patterns clear but do not exaggerate or over-emphasize your speech.

- Speak a little louder if necessary but don't shout, as this distorts your lip patterns (AND IT'S RUDE!)

- Use body language, gestures, and facial expressions to help your verbal communication.

- Allow extra time and be patient. Communicating with a deaf or hard-of-hearing person can be hard work for both of you – if the deaf person gets tired, stop.

If you are not making yourself understood

- Be aware that just because a person is smiling and nodding, it does not necessarily mean they understand you.

- Similarly, you should not pretend to have understood if you have not – clarify and check.

- If you have not made yourself understood the first time, repeat key phrases, and if this does not work try rephrasing the whole sentence using different words, as some words are easier to lip-read than others.

- Writing down key words or drawing diagrams is also a good way to clarify.

Communication issues for blind and partially sighted people

Remember that people who cannot see you will not be able to pick up on any of the subtleties of your non-verbal communication. You will need to verbalize everything, and describe everything out loud. In addition, when you enter a room, you need to let the person know you are there – approach them from the front and introduce yourself and anyone else who is there. Similarly, when you leave, you need to say that you are going, or you risk letting the person carry on talking to empty space. When you are guiding someone who is blind or partially sighted, ask them what kind of help they want from you. If they want you to guide them, offer them your elbow or gently place their hand on your elbow – do not grab them or 'manhandle' them. Remember to describe any obstacles such as

approaching steps. For people who have some residual vision, remember to make sure there is sufficient light in the room. Finally, if a blind person has a guide dog, remember that the dog is working, and stroking it will distract it, so ask the owner's permission first.

Talking with people who are deafblind

A person is regarded as deafblind when they have a visual and hearing impairment, and when the combination of both intensifies the impact of the other, thus preventing them functioning as a blind person who can hear or as a deaf person who can see (Hicks, 2006). Deafblindness is a relatively rare disability, although it is more common in environments such as audiology and ophthalmology settings. Many healthcare professionals' lack of experience, knowledge, or skills in communicating with deafblind people often leads to fear and withdrawal, and deafblind people commonly experience simply being left alone, which increases their isolation (Sense and Deafblind UK, 2001).

Deafblind people use a variety of communication methods, although most will continue to use speech, provided it is a little slower and clearer than usual speech. Some deafblind people use the deafblind manual alphabet to communicate, which is an alphabet with a sign for each letter. With the exception of a few letters, the deafblind manual alphabet is the same as the deaf alphabet. If a person does use the deafblind manual alphabet to communicate, they will need to have an appropriate interpreter booked, as well as a double appointment. Another way to communicate with a deafblind person is by using block alphabet, which involves spelling out letters on a person's hand.

TIPS ON COMMUNICATING WITH A PERSON WHO IS DEAFBLIND

Most of the tips above on communicating with people who are hearing or visually impaired are also relevant to deafblind people. In addition:

- Try addressing the person by name – they may be able to hear speech or sounds

- Write notes:
  - Use a black felt-tip pen on white paper
  - Check with the person how large the letters should be
  - Leave ample spaces between lines and at the end of words
  - Write neatly with full punctuation
  - Keep sentences short

◆ Use block alphabet – a manual form of communication where words are spelled out on to the palm of the deafblind person's hand:
  - Trace each letter with your finger, in block capitals, on the palm
  - Use the whole of the palm for each letter
  - Keep letters large and clear
  - Place one letter on top of the last
  - Pause slightly at the end of each word (Hicks, 2006)

◆ Use textphone services
  - There are various technologies available where messages are typed by the deafblind person, and an operator reads them out to you. You reply in the normal way (speaking slightly slowly) so that the operator has time to type out what you are saying.

There is more information about how to communicate with someone who is deafblind, including diagrams of the deafblind alphabet, on the SENSE charity website, the link to which is available via the Online Resource Centre associated with this book.

Talking with people with learning disabilities

The term 'learning disability' covers a very wide spectrum of intellectual impairment. At one end of that spectrum are people who have no particular communication needs over and above those of all patients. When talking with people with a mild learning disability, as with all patients, you should remember to (Byron *et al.*, 2006):

◆ give information in manageable 'chunks'

◆ ask them to repeat back to check understanding

◆ avoid medical jargon

◆ not let supporters/carers answer questions for the person unless the disabled person has asked them for their help

◆ explain clearly and simply what will happen before you take any action.

At the other end of the spectrum of learning disabilities are those people who have profound and multiple learning disabilities (PMLD). While people with less severe learning disabilities may be able to communicate using techniques such as short sentences and appropriate pictures or technical support, people with PMLD may have little or no expression or understanding of language; they may also have physical or sensory disabilities, severely impaired intellectual and social

functioning, associated medical conditions, and may need constant support and supervision. Therefore, people with PMLD cannot use formal methods of communication such as speech, signing, writing, or symbols. These people may communicate in their own unique way using their bodies, facial expressions, sounds, reflex responses, actions, eye gaze, or pointing, and it can be difficult to interpret these signals.

People with PMLD may attempt to exercise control over their lives verbally or non-verbally by refusing an activity proposed by supporters: edging away from an activity, turning their head away, standing facing the wall, standing still when encouraged to approach, or by the use of shrieks or sounds such as 'nehr' (Finlay *et al.*, 2008). This may often be interpreted as 'challenging behaviour', for example **'He spits out his food on purpose'** (Thurman *et al.*, 2005). Research indicates that up to 45% of people with an intellectual disability in hospital and up to 20% in the community are on antipsychotic drugs for challenging behaviours (Regnard *et al.*, 2007).

When you meet a person with PMLD it is important to talk with the most significant people in their lives, as they will be your source of information about ways to communicate with them: their family and people with whom the person comes into contact daily, their teachers, escorts, and speech and language therapists for example. Include the person with PMLD in the discussion by talking to their significant others in their presence. Ask how well they can see or hear, about their range of movements – are they able to orientate their body away or point to something, for example? How do they express pain and distress? Also ask about their general level of health, and how this might affect the consistency of their responses (Porter *et al.*, 2001).

QUESTIONS TO ASK THE SIGNIFICANT OTHERS OF A PERSON WITH PMLD

◆ How do you communicate with them?

◆ What do you think they understand in different situations?

◆ What difficulties, if any, do you encounter in communicating with them?

◆ How do you support their communication?

◆ How can you be certain of your interpretation of their communication?

Porter *et al.* (2001)

One particular difficulty lies in telling whether or not a person with PMLD is in pain or whether they are distressed by something else. An increase in activity due to distress may be misinterpreted as challenging behaviour or as the person being in pain. If distress is misdiagnosed as pain, then the resulting sedation from analgesia can reinforce the misapprehension that the patient was in pain in the first place. Distress can be identified in people with little or no verbal communication by observing changes in their behaviour, posture, or most commonly through their facial expression or through autonomic skin changes such as flushed skin or sweating. Distress is usually associated with new behaviours, or a change from the norm, and again here you need to ask the person's significant others' opinions (Regnard *et al.*, 2007).

SIGNS AND BEHAVIOURS INDICATING PAIN OR DISTRESS IN PEOPLE WITH INTELLECTUAL DISABILITY

This includes people with PMLD, but also people in the later stages of dementia, severely ill patients, and so on:

♦ Facial expression, absence of contentment

♦ Withdrawal, refusing food, changes in habits or mannerisms

♦ Aggression, agitation, increased body movement

♦ Moaning, sighing, noisy breathing

♦ Wincing, grimacing, crying, changes in vocalization

♦ Guarding, bracing, rigidity, holding head, protecting limb

♦ Fidgeting, repetitive vocalization

♦ Changes in skin colour, sweating, increase in blood pressure or pulse

Regnard *et al.* (2007)

Summary

As a medical student and doctor, you will encounter many disabled people. For some of these people, their impairment will result in difficulties in communicating, while for others, it will affect other aspects of their lives. The doctor's role in helping disabled people is not to provide a 'cure' – their 'problems' do not have medical 'solutions'. The doctor's role, and legal duty, is to provide access to the same quality of healthcare as other patients, and not to allow assumptions or prejudices relating to disability to affect this adversely. Doctors should diagnose any complications or the causes of any changes in disabled peoples' abilities, help to treat any symptoms they have such as pain, provide expertise on recent medical advances, and provide access to other professionals and organizations that can provide help (The Disability Partnership, 2000). Remember that the real experts on disability are disabled people themselves.

Further reading

A. Kvalsvig is a deaf doctor, whose perspective on disability is interesting and thought provoking.

Kvalsvig, A. (2003). Ask the elephant. *The Lancet* **362** (9401): 2079–2080.

One of the best sources of up-to-date information on all disabilities is from the various charities' websites, and this chapter is indebted to many of them. There are links to many more of the disability charities' websites available via the Online Resource Centre for this book.

Visit the Online Resource Centre for *Clinical Communication Skills* at: www.oxfordtextbooks.co.uk/orc/washer

References

Byron, M., Howell, C., Bradley, P., Bheenuck, S., Wickham, C., and Curran, T. (2006). *Different Differences: Disability Equality Teaching in Healthcare Education.* Bristol: University of Bristol, University of the West of England, and Peninsula Medical School.

Dalton, P. (1994). *Counselling People with Communication Problems.* London: Sage Publications.

Finlay, W., Antaki, C., and Walton, C. (2008). Saying no to the staff: An analysis of refusals in a home for people with severe communication difficulties. *Sociology of Health and Illness*, **30**(1), 55–75.

Hearing Concern (2006a). *Deaf Awareness – Terminology.* London: Hearing Concern.

Hearing Concern (2006b). *Top Ten Communication Tips to Remember When You Talk to People Who are Hard of Hearing.* London: Hearing Concern.

Hicks, G. (2006). *Making Contact – A Good Practice Guide: How to Involve and Communicate With a Deafblind Person.* London: Sense.

Miller, P., Parker, S., and Gillinson, S. (2004). *Disablism: How to Tackle the Last Prejudice.* London: Demos.

National Institute on Deafness and Other Communication Disorders (1997). *Aphasia.* Bethesda, MD, USA: National Institute on Deafness and Other Communication Disorders.

Porter, J., Ouvry, C., Morgan, M., and Downs, C. (2001). Interpreting the communication of people with profound and multiple learning difficulties. *British Journal of Learning Disabilities*, **29**, 12–16.

Regnard, C., Reynolds, J., Watson, B., Matthews, D., Gibson, L., and Clarke, C. (2007). Understanding distress in people with severe communication difficulties: Developing and assessing the Disability Distress Assessment Tool (DisDAT). *Journal of Intellectual Disability Research*, **51**(4), 277–292.

RNID (2006). Communication tips for hearing people. London: Royal National Institute of the Deaf.

Sense (2003). *How Do People Who Are Deafblind Communicate?* London: Sense.

Sense (2006). *Communicating With Your Deafblind Patients.* London: Sense.

Sense and Deafblind UK (2001). *Who Cares? Access to Healthcare for Deafblind People.* London: Sense and Deafblind UK.

The Disability Partnership (2000). *One in Four of Us: The Experience of Disability.* London: The Disability Partnership.

Thurman, S., Jones, J., and Tarleton, B. (2005). Without words – meaningful information for people with high individual communication needs. *British Journal of Learning Disabilities*, **33**, 83–89.

CHAPTER 8

Talking with people from other cultures

Peter Washer

Learning points

This chapter will:

◆ help you reflect on your own cultural background

◆ examine the effects of culture on clinical communication

◆ discuss strategies for dealing with prejudice and racism

◆ describe best practice when talking with patients and their families who speak English as an additional language, as well as in working with interpreters.

Often when people talk about 'culture' – the customs and institutions of a particular group of people – they only think in terms of black and minority ethnic (BME) people. However, culture is not something that only *other people* have. We are all the products of a distinct and unique culture, whether we ascribe to our own culture's values or not. It is easy to be blind to the influence of your own culture, and to see your own world view as 'universal', 'natural', or 'taken for granted' in comparison with the views of other cultures, which by comparison seem exotic, strange, or bizarre.

Miner (1956), writing in the journal *American Anthropologist*, described a tribe called the 'Nacirema', who lived in the territory between the Canadian Cree, the Yaqui and Tarahumare of Mexico, and the Carib and Arawak of the Antilles.

BODY RITUAL AMONG THE NACIREMA

Underlying the whole Nacirema system of beliefs was their conception of the human body as ugly and having a natural tendency to debility and disease. The only hope of diverting these characteristics was through ritual and ceremonies using charms and magical potions. These were secured from a variety of specialized practitioners, the most powerful of which were the medicine men, whose assistance was rewarded with substantial gifts. In every community, the medicine men had an imposing temple – a *latipso* – where the more elaborate ceremonies required to treat very sick people, such as jabbing magically treated needles into their flesh, were performed. These ceremonies involved a permanent group of Vestal maidens who moved sedately about the temple in distinctive costume and headdress. The ceremonies performed in the *latipso* were so harsh that only a proportion of the supplicants entering the temple ever recovered, although this in no way decreased the people's faith in the medicine men.

Miner (1956)

Some readers will already have guessed that Miner's account is actually a spoof: *nacirema* is American spelt backwards, and the *latipso* is an 'ospital. Given its medical context, this elaborate joke alerts us to how bizarre and unfathomable the customs and beliefs of any culture can seem from the outside.

Your own cultural background

If someone were to ask you, **'What's your cultural background?'**, what would be the first thing that came into your mind? What sorts of things are valued by your culture, at least by the mainstream of opinion within it? For example, does your culture value independence and self-help, or are extended family ties and inheritance more important? Does your culture value youth, or is there deference to elders or authority figures? Does competition and future-thinking dominate the way you think about the world (think about your exams to get into medical school!), or is the past more important? Does spirituality or religion play a part in the way your cultural group lives, or are materialism and individualism more important? What holidays do you observe in your culture? What foods do you eat? Food is a good example of something that is distinctive to a particular culture, and of course there are widely different attitudes to alcohol across cultures.

Usually, when people talk about 'my culture' they either mean their religion or their ethnic background. Sometimes they might mean their social class or some other influence such as their nationality that they feel is important. In a multicultural society, many people have a mix of cultural influences, and will negotiate their way between the mainstream culture and the culture of their family background. However, families and individuals are all different, and *within* a cultural group there will be as much diversity as there is *between* different cultural groups. For example, it does not follow that because you are a member of a particular ethnic group you will necessarily be rich or poor, educated or uneducated, religious or secular.

Although the word 'race' is often used as a synonym for ethnicity, historical ideas about race that conceive biologically determined 'racial' differences between human populations are now discredited. All human beings belong to the same species; the differences between us are cultural. Ethnicity means identifying with a social group not only because you may have different physical features, as in 'race', but more importantly because you identify with the culture of that group, for example 'black British', 'British Asian', 'African–American', and so on.

Cultural awareness teaching in medical schools has been criticized for its superficial descriptions of the different prevalence of disease in specific cultural groups, or because it focuses on describing different cultural beliefs or practices (Kai *et al.*, 2006b). This approach risks underlining stereotypes we may already have, and it would anyway be impossible to learn about all the different cultures you might possibly encounter. Instead, we need to learn how to ask appropriate questions to obtain information about the individual patient's culture, and to be 'culturally aware' – to view individuals in their cultural context and take note of other influences on their health, such as socioeconomic influences and social inequalities.

Although most research on cross-cultural communication defines 'culture' in terms of ethnicity, there is some research evidence that points to the importance of class-based barriers to communication. For example, one US study of 336 outpatient consultations found that patients from upper-middle-class backgrounds received more doctor time and more explanations than patients from lower-middle-class or working-class backgrounds (Waitzkin, 1985). This effect is likely to be even greater in a more class-conscious society such as Britain, but in any country, there is always going to be a communication gap between doctors and most of their patients in terms of social class. Whatever your class background on entering medical school, by the time you leave it you will be better educated, better paid, and have higher social status – and thus be more powerful – than most of your patients. This aspect of cross-cultural communication is less often addressed than communication across ethnic groups, but is no less likely to be a barrier to understanding.

The other thing to say about culture is that although customs and traditions may appear ancient and unchanging, cultures are continually transforming and reinterpreting themselves, often quite rapidly. These changes are driven and influenced by powerful societal forces such as politics and the mass media.

The effects of culture on clinical communication

Why is all this important for medical students? Firstly, because the world is becoming increasingly globalized, and histories of mass migration mean that just about all doctors, wherever they practise, will have culturally diverse patient populations. Within and across the ethnic groups, nationalities, and religions, there may be subcultures grouped around lines such as social class, sexuality, age, and so on. While some of these distinctions are visible, others may be less so.

Secondly, learning to talk with people from other cultures is important because research indicates that it is often done badly. For example, a review of the literature on cross-cultural communication found that doctors related to their BME patients differently; they were less friendly and concerned with BME patients, there was less social talk and rapport building, and they were more likely to ignore their comments (Schouten & Meeuwesen, 2006). Similarly, a review of US-based research also found that ethnicity had a substantial influence on the quality of the doctor–patient relationship. BME patients, particularly those not proficient in English, were less likely to engender empathic responses from doctors, to receive sufficient information, and to be encouraged to participate in medical decision making (Ferguson & Candib, 2002).

Culture can be an important influencing factor in doctor–patient communication in a number of respects. Patients may not share the same world view as their doctor, and there may be different expectations of the doctor–patient relationship. The rest of this section will expand on these aspects of the effects of culture.

Non-Western medicine

Just as food is culturally specific, Western medicine is itself a product of Western culture, has its own specific language, and is associated with a specific power position (Surbone, 2008). Western medicine has culturally derived notions of health, disease – what doctors diagnose – and illness – what patients experience. In the Western biomedical model, a patient's symptoms must be 'caused' by some underlying 'disease' or else they are not 'real' – see Chapter 12 in this book for a further exploration of this issue.

However, in some cultures, explanations for illnesses may be religious or spiritual, for example, that the sick are being punished for having done something wrong. Sometimes patients might attribute their problems to the 'evil eye' or express fatalism that their illness is 'God's will'. They may also hide these beliefs from their doctors for fear of ridicule, and as a result not adhere to their Western medical treatment (Hudelson, 2005). If all this sounds strange or backward to you, think about how, even in Western culture, many people believe that cancer is the expression or the result of some unresolved psychological issue – 'eating away at you like a cancer' – and afflicts people who are sexually repressed, inhibited, lacking spontaneity, or incapable of expressing passion or anger. Another widely held belief in Western culture is that AIDS is 'nature's revenge' (for the secular) or 'God's punishment' (for the religious) for homosexuality and promiscuity. For a fascinating exploration of these issues, see Susan Sontag's famous essays *Illness as Metaphor* and *AIDS and its Metaphors* (Sontag, 1978, 1989).

Some cultures have ancient and developed systems of medicine that are rooted in entirely different paradigms to Western notions of scientific experiment and rational materialism, for example Traditional Chinese Medicine (TCM) or Ayurvedic medicine. In these different systems, there may be notions of blood being too 'hot' or 'cold', 'thin', 'thick', or 'stagnant'. The cure for symptoms caused by these underlying problems may be to eat certain foods, to keep warm, and so on. If a Western doctor prescribes treatment or gives advice that conflicts with these notions, then adherence to that treatment plan may be poor. For example, research among Chinese and Vietnamese-American patients found that they used TCM before seeking Western medical care, and while they wanted to discuss their beliefs and practices with their Western doctors, they were reluctant to do so as they often encountered negative and judgemental responses. Sometimes TCM practices such as 'coining', where the spine and sternum are rubbed with oil and a coin to release the 'wind' or 'cold'; and 'cupping', where air is heated in a cup and placed onto the skin to 'pull out the cold air' were mistaken by their Western doctors as signs of haematological diseases or abuse (Ngo-Metzger *et al.*, 2003).

The doctor's expectations of the patient and family

As well as in the form of different beliefs about causation and cure, culture can impact on doctor–patient communication in terms of different expectations of roles, both from the doctor's perspective and from that of the patient and their family. In the West, doctors expect to deal with individual patients, whereas in some cultures the whole family will expect to be involved in making medical decisions. Western medicine (and nursing) promotes independence and self-caring as a virtue, but this may conflict with notions that the extended family should care for their own sick and old people. In some cultures, it would be considered shameful that old or sick relatives should care for themselves or should be cared for by strangers.

In comparison with Western openness about sex and sexuality, other cultures may be more sensitive to discussing sexual matters. There is an assumption that certain cultural groups, particularly Asian women, have a preference for seeing a female doctor. However, research suggests that both white and Asian women patients prefer female doctors when discussing 'women's problems' (Ali *et al.*, 2006). Incidentally, although female patients are often given consideration in this respect, male patients of any cultural background are rarely given the same courtesy, yet it may be the case that many male patients may prefer a male doctor when discussing embarrassing problems such as impotence, incontinence, and so on.

The patient's expectations of the doctor

While doctors may have certain culturally specific expectations of their patients, patients' expectations of doctors may similarly be culturally bound. In cultures where there is more deference to authority figures or 'experts' than there is today in the West, patients may not expect to have the relationship of partnership with their doctors that most Western patients expect. However, research in developing countries suggests that, as in developed countries, patient-centred models of communication are likely to produce better outcomes than doctor-centred models. For example, one Egyptian study found that women were more likely to be satisfied with the consultation and continue using a particular contraceptive method if the consultation was patient-centred, and were less likely to continue using

the method if the doctor was negative or directive (Abdel-Tawab & Roter, 2002). Although some aspects of patient expectations are therefore likely to be culturally specific, some elements of patient preferences, such as the need to be heard and understood, are likely to be universal (Schouten & Meeuwesen, 2006).

BEST PRACTICE WHEN COMMUNICATING WITH PEOPLE FROM OTHER CULTURES

- Explore cultural issues and practices sensitively but directly and do not be afraid to ask about cultural issues when appropriate.

- Acknowledge that cultural issues are important and show respect for the beliefs of others.

- Explain why you are asking about cultural issues; in other words, make sure it is clear to the patient how your questions are relevant to their care.

- Be sensitive to cultural differences:
  - in terms of non-verbal communication – whether to shake hands, maintain eye contact, and so on
  - in terms of verbal cues – conventions of politeness, mode of address, indirectness, and so on.

- Be aware that your own (Western medical) ideas about health, disease, and illness are as culturally specific as your patients'.

- Try to avoid the notion that your own culture is any more 'natural' or 'normal' than other 'strange' cultures.

- Don't pretend you know about some cultural practice or belief if you do not.

- Remember that patients may expect you to be unsympathetic to their cultural beliefs or their use of other medical systems, so you need to explore these proactively, rather than waiting to be told.

- Remember that even if you know a particular culture well, it does not follow that this person will be a 'typical' example.

Finally, if you do encounter a situation where a patient says that their culture or their religious beliefs forbid them consenting to something, for example having a blood transfusion or giving consent for a postmortem, then ask them if you can contact a leader of their religion or community. Organize a meeting with them together with the patient and family. The religious leader will have more authority in the eyes of the patient and is likely to know if there are any ways to accommodate the situation within the bounds of their shared belief system.

Strategies for dealing with prejudice and racism

Racism is prejudice or discrimination based on ideas about 'race'. This can be expressed individually, in the context of prejudice or stereotyping people based on notions of the supposed superiority or inferiority of individuals with certain 'racial' characteristics. Racism can also be expressed through institutional policies or practices, which is sometimes called 'institutional racism'. For example, after the botched investigation into the racist murder of black teenager Stephen Lawrence in London in 1993, an inquiry dubbed the Metropolitan Police 'institutionally racist'. A similar charge has been made against healthcare institutions' policies and practices.

One common problem that medical students and doctors face is in dealing with patients who are racially prejudiced. BME doctors and other health professionals are often subject to racial discrimination from their patients and colleagues, as are white foreign doctors. For example, the UK Department of Health commissioned focus group research with 494 BME staff working in the National Health Service and found that 46.2% of them had experienced racial harassment, and 37.9% had witnessed racial harassment at work in the previous 12 months. This was most commonly verbal abuse from patients, or patients refusing care from BME staff, and most instances went unreported (Lemos & Crane, 2000). Patients and staff often perceive BME doctors and nurses as less well qualified, less competent, and less well trained. Research suggests that students also encounter patients who are racist to professionals (Kai *et al.*, 2006a). Dealing with racist behaviour patients is not only an issue for BME staff. Often patients will make racist remarks to white doctors and nurses when they think it is 'safe' to do so.

If a patient or another member of staff racially harasses you, another member of staff or another patient, you should report the incident. Each hospital or Trust will have a written policy on racial harassment and a system for recording and dealing with such matters. You should seek advice about who you should report the incident to, as there will be someone with designated responsibility for this.

However, most incidents of racial prejudice from patients are not that clear-cut and it is often the 'grey' areas that cause dilemmas. For example, a patient may complain of a bad experience they had from a previous doctor of a particular BME group and ask if they can see a white doctor. Patients will often make this kind of request even to BME doctors or nurses, with a caveat that 'you're not like that'. There's no single 'correct' response in these situations. There is a complicated dilemma here of balancing a patient's autonomy to prefer to see someone from a similar background, yet not colluding with racial or other types of prejudice. Different types of intervention are required to address different forms of racism (Gunaratnam, 2001). In these circumstances, it is up to your professional judgement to decide how to react. However, you need to remember that if you do not deal with the situation at all, then you risk being seen as colluding with the patient, who may presume that you are as prejudiced as they are.

SOME POSSIBLE STRATEGIES FOR DEALING WITH RACIALLY PREJUDICED PATIENTS

- Use non-verbal signals to show your displeasure (all the things you have been taught NOT to do in other circumstances) – lose eye contact, don't smile, look bored, and use your hand(s) to indicate STOP!

- Pointedly redirect the conversation and change the subject.

- Personalize when patients generalize – for example, if a patient makes a general pejorative comment about Asian doctors, look them straight in the eye and say **'Dr Shah is a really good doctor.'**

- Be prepared to rephrase patients' use of language if it offends you. For example, if a patient says **'I saw a coloured doctor last time'**, when you reflect that back to them, say, **'You said you saw a black doctor . . .'**

- Remember you don't have to laugh if you do not find something funny.

- Try not to show the patient that you are angry or raise your voice.

- Do not respond positively to any cues that you think might be racist.

- Avoid colluding with the patient if they are being racist.

- Silence can be very powerful.

Patients who have English as an additional language

One of the more obvious barriers to communicating with people from other cultures is that many patients you will encounter will not speak English very well. In London, for example, there are up to 340 languages spoken, and an estimated 5–25% of consultations with GPs either involve an interpreter or are compromised for the lack of one. This is especially true for refugees and asylum seekers, many of whom have complex, serious, and stigmatizing conditions, such as mental health problems or HIV, or have come from war zones where they have suffered trauma and rape (Greenhalgh *et al.*, 2007).

When patients have limited English, remember your key communication skills:

- give information in manageable chunks and check they have understood as you go

- watch the patient carefully and be aware of their non-verbal cues

- deal with one topic at a time

- signpost

- avoid jargon

- use diagrams and written material.

One particular strategy is to allow patients with limited English to continue speaking even when they seem to be straying away off topic. Research shows that, by producing a narrative in their own terms and without the burden of answering a stream of questions, patients with limited English are freed to tell their stories in a way in which they feel competent, concentrating on their emotional state and not on the distraction of having to process the English language (Moss & Roberts, 2005).

Best practice in using interpreters

When a patient does not speak English at all, or where their English is not of a standard to safely continue a medical consultation with them, you will need to use an interpreter. Ideally, this should be a trained medical interpreter, either in person or over the telephone. However, necessity often dictates that friends of the patient or members of their family, often their children, act as interpreters. Using family members to interpret is far from ideal, as it may lead to reluctance to discuss sensitive issues, there may be mistranslation, there may be hidden family tensions, and if the interpreter is a child, they may not be sufficiently mature to

effectively interpret what is going on. Sometimes a bilingual health professional can interpret if necessary, but this can also lead to a problem of blurring of professional boundaries.

Ideally, a professional interpreter will be more effective, can offer cultural insights, can correctly interpret medical terms, and will help facilitate a better management plan. However, even with a professional interpreter, there may still be issues that can cause problems. Tensions may arise if they are from a different social class, ethnic group, or gender to the patient. This can be particularly problematic for asylum seekers, who may be faced with an interpreter from the same group that they have been oppressed by in their country of origin. Therefore, it is important to match patients and interpreters carefully. Patients may also feel reluctant to discuss private matters in front of a stranger who is not a doctor, and the patient may have concerns about confidentiality, particularly if both patient and interpreter are from a small community.

Even when using a professional interpreter, you should be careful that they are acting as a conduit and not covertly editing patients' and healthcare professionals' speech. For example, one US study examined the practice of 26 professional interpreters and found that at times they over-stepped the boundaries of their role. For example, they would decide that the patient's answer was not complete and initiate information re-seeking they felt was necessary on behalf of the healthcare professional, or they would try to bridge cultural differences by using Western biomedical concepts to replace the patient's culturally specific comments such as **'I caught the wind'**, which would be translated as **'She's got a cold.'** Although the interpreters claimed they did not provide medical information to the patients, observations suggested they did, and the patient was not in a position to know that the information had come from the interpreter rather than the healthcare professional (Hsieh, 2007).

Another Swiss study explored the perspectives of nine professional medical interpreters who described misunderstandings they had encountered between doctors and patients; for example, patients often experienced a psychological diagnosis as rejection and disbelief on the part of the doctor. Some diagnoses were particularly stigmatizing, such as tuberculosis or forms of mental illness, and as a result some patients rejected the diagnosis or tried to hide the disease. Another area where there was misunderstanding was when, for example, patients felt uncomfortable when doctors asked them questions about their personal life. For the doctors, these were standard questions, but patients perceived them as inappropriate and intrusive in the context of a medical consultation as they reminded them of interviews with immigration officials. Finally, misunderstandings followed from differences in communication styles, where gestures, eye contact, and vocabulary meant different things for doctors and patients (Hudelson, 2005).

WORKING WELL WITH AN INTERPRETER

Practical things to do:

- Check that the interpreter and the patient speak the same language and the same dialect.
- Allow time for pre-interview discussion with the interpreter in order to talk about the contents of the interview and the way in which you will work together.
- Ask the interpreter to teach you how to pronounce the patient's name correctly.
- Allow time for the interpreter to:
  - introduce themselves to the patient and explain their role
  - explain that the interview will be kept confidential
  - check whether they are an acceptable interpreter for the patient
  - introduce you and your role to the patient.
- Encourage the interpreter to interrupt and intervene during the consultation as necessary.
- Use straightforward language and avoid jargon.
- Actively listen to the interpreter and the patient.
- Maintain more eye contact with the patient to offset the chances of the primary relationship being between the interpreter and the patient.
- Allow enough time for the interview, perhaps double the time you might allocate for an English-speaking patient. Incidentally, a consultation with a patient with limited English without an interpreter may take just as long.
- At the end of the interview, check that the patient has understood everything or whether they want to ask anything else.
- Have a post-interview discussion with the interpreter if appropriate.

From Kai (1999)

Summary

Culture – both yours and the patient's – will influence medical communication and it is important to be aware of those influences and acknowledge them. Treat people as individuals, but at the same time acknowledge the influence of culture and explore it when you feel it is relevant and necessary. Do not be afraid to tackle issues around race and culture, including racism. Finally, when patients have limited English, use interpreting services where available, but be aware of the complexities of this type of three-way conversation.

Further reading

This chapter has focused on patients who have limited English, but any medical students or doctors who need to improve their English should see:

Glendinning, E.H. and Holmstrom, B.A.S. (2005) *English in Medicine*, 3rd edn. Cambridge: Cambridge University Press.

Visit the Online Resource Centre for *Clinical Communication Skills* at: www.oxfordtextbooks.co.uk/orc/washer

References

Abdel-Tawab, N. and Roter, D. (2002). The relevance of client-centered communication to family planning settings in developing countries: Lessons from the Egyptian experience. *Social Science and Medicine*, **54**(9), 1357–1368.

Ali, N., Atkin, K., and Neal, R. (2006). The role of culture in the general practice consultation process. *Ethnicity and Health*, **11**(4), 389–408.

Ferguson, W.J. and Candib, L.M. (2002). Culture, language, and the doctor–patient relationship. *Family Medicine*, **34**(5), 353–361.

Greenhalgh, T., Voisey, C., and Robb, N. (2007). Interpreted consultations as 'business as usual'? An analysis of organisational routines in general practices. *Sociology of Health and Illness*, **29**(6), 931–954.

Gunaratnam, Y. (2001). 'We mustn't judge people ... but': Staff dilemmas in dealing with racial harassment amongst hospice service users. *Sociology of Health and Illness*, **23**(1), 65–84.

Hsieh, E. (2007). Interpreters as co-diagnosticians: Overlapping roles and services between providers and interpreters. *Social Science and Medicine*, **64**, 924–937.

Hudelson, P. (2005). Improving patient–provider communication: Insights from interpreters. *Family Practice*, **22**(3), 311–316.

Kai, J. (1999). *Valuing Diversity: A Resource for Effective Health Care of Ethnically Diverse Communities*. London: The Royal College of General Practitioners.

Kai, J., Bridgewater, R., and Spencer, J. (2006a). 'Just think of TB and Asians, that's all I ever hear': Medical learners' views about training to work in an ethnically diverse society. *Medical Education*, **35**(3), 250–256.

Kai, J., Spencer, J., and Woodward, N. (2006b). Wrestling with ethnic diversity: Toward empowering health educators. *Medical Education*, **35**(3), 262–271.

Lemos, P. and Crane, G. (2000). *Tackling Racial Harassment in the NHS: Evaluating Black and Minority Ehnic Staff's Atitudes and Experiences*. London: Department of Health.

Miner, H. (1956). Body ritual among the Nacirema. *American Anthropologist*, **58**(3), 503–507.

Moss, B. and Roberts, C. (2005). Explanations, explanations, explanations: How do patients with limited English construct narrative accounts in multi-lingual, multi-ethnic settings, and how can GPs interpret them? *Family Practice*, **22**(4), 412–418.

Ngo-Metzger, Q., Massagli, M.P., Clarridge, B.R., Manocchia, M., Davis, R.B., Iezzoni, L.I., and Phillips, R.S. (2003). Linguistic and cultural barriers to care. *Journal of General Internal Medicine*, **18**(1), 44–52.

Schouten, B.C. and Meeuwesen, L. (2006). Cultural differences in medical communication: A review of the literature. *Patient Education and Counselling*, **64**, 21–34.

Sontag, S. (1978). *Illness as Metaphor*. London: Penguin Books.

Sontag, S. (1989). *AIDS and its Metaphors*. USA: Farra, Straus & Giroux.

Surbone, A. (2008). Cultural aspects of communication in cancer care. *Support Cancer Care*, **16**, 235–240.

Waitzkin, H. (1985). Information giving in medical care. *Journal of Health and Social Behavior*, **26**(2), 81–101.

CHAPTER 9

Talking about sex and sexuality

Peter Washer

Learning points

This chapter will:

- identify when doctors need to talk about sex and sexuality with patients
- reflect on how doctors' attitudes can impact on their ability to discuss sex and sexuality
- discuss the needs of lesbian, gay, bisexual, and transgender patients (and health professionals)
- describe when and how you might need to talk about sex in more detail.

Sex and sexuality are fundamental aspects of human identity and impact on all aspects of our lives, so it is important that healthcare professionals are able to talk confidently about them. Many people find it difficult to talk about sex and sexuality, including many medical students and doctors. Often, how to talk about sexual matters is taught in relation to genitourinary medicine, or to obstetrics and gynaecology. While this is understandable, it reinforces the misapprehension that sex and sexuality are only an issue when the problem is obviously related to 'sexual health'. This chapter will examine the issues around talking about sex and sexuality, and discuss when doctors and patients might need to talk about sex in a broader context.

When might we need to talk about sex and sexuality?

When the problem is obviously related to sex

Doctors and patients need to talk frankly about sexual matters when patients present with a sexually transmitted infection or when they seek advice relating to issues like HIV. Talking about sex is also an essential part of history taking with women who have gynaecological problems or when they need routine cervical screening, when patients seek advice about conception, contraception, pregnancy, and abortion, and in caring for victims of rape or abuse.

Sexual consequences of medical and surgical conditions

As well as 'sexual health' problems, most common medical and surgical conditions may also impact on a person's physical ability to have or to enjoy sex, and patients may wish to discuss this with their doctor. Some examples might be:

◆ patients with cardiac or lung disease, for example following myocardial infarction

◆ patients with limited mobility, for example following a cerebrovascular accident (stroke) or due to a medical condition such as multiple sclerosis

◆ men with diabetes who can suffer with erectile dysfunction (the inability to develop and maintain an erection for satisfactory sexual activity)

◆ patients suffering pain, for example due to some underlying condition like arthritis.

One common side effect of many medicines is that they can lead to sexual problems, such as decreasing sexual desire or arousal. Recreational drugs like cannabis and alcohol can initially decrease inhibitions and increase sexual confidence, but both can affect people's (particularly men's) ability to have sex. In other words, most common medical conditions can affect patients' sex lives in various ways, and therefore outside of obvious 'sexual health' contexts, patients might need or want to talk about sex with their doctor at some time.

Sexual problems related to psychosocial issues

As well as these physical problems, psychosocial problems can lead to problems with sexual desire, arousal, or orgasm. Patients with altered body image following an accident or surgery, such as amputees, people who are scarred, women following mastectomy, or people with a colostomy for example, may feel less sexually attractive or desirable. Patients who are depressed may suffer from a reduced desire to have sex. Patients suffering from mental illness may be sexually disinhibited. People with a history of sexual abuse or rape may have problems enjoying sex. There are also the more everyday features of modern life, such as tiredness, overwork, and stress, which can cause relationship problems, or lead to an inability or lack of energy to enjoy sex.

What is 'sexual health'?

By broadening the scope of the discussion of when doctors and patients need to talk about sex away from strictly speaking 'sexual' problems, we can see that 'sexual health' (like mental health) involves more than just the absence of disease. The following definition of sexual health was proposed by an international consultation of sexual health experts convened by the World Health Organization:

'Sexual health is a state of physical, emotional, mental and social well-being in relation to sexuality; it is not merely the absence of disease, dysfunction or infirmity. Sexual health requires a positive and respectful approach to sexuality and sexual relationships, as well as the possibility of having pleasurable and safe sexual experiences, free of coercion, discrimination and violence. For sexual health to be attained and maintained, the sexual rights of all persons must be respected, protected and fulfilled' (WHO, 2002).

Doctors' attitudes to sex and sexuality

Medical schools have historically given little attention to sexuality, and perhaps as a consequence, doctors often have little confidence or feel embarrassed discussing it (Bonvicini & Perlin, 2003). Research shows that medical students' and doctors' knowledge about issues relating to sexuality is often poor and that they often do not deal with sexuality well. For example, one web-based survey of 208 students in an English medical school found that there was poor knowledge of sexual health issues such as the failure rate of condoms, abortion rates, and the prevalence of *Chlamydia* (Fayers et al., 2003). Another Australian survey of 576 medical and nursing students found a significant relationship between those who were religious (of any religion) and negative attitudes to homosexuality, masturbation, premarital sex, and contraception. Some students also absented themselves from lectures where such material was discussed, suggesting that their attitudes may well have resulted in discriminatory practice with patients (McKelvey *et al.*, 1999).

Research suggests that, once qualified, doctors are also often less than comfortable in discussing sex and sexuality with patients. For example, one Belgian study surveyed 122 GPs and found that about half of them failed to counsel an asymptomatic patient with an obvious sexually transmitted infection risk, and as many again gave no safer-sex advice in a first contraceptive consultation. The GPs cited barriers to these discussions such as language and comprehension problems, ethnic differences, insufficient training, lack of time, presence of the patient's partner or parent, that the patient had no genital complaints, and fear of embarrassing the patient (Verhoeven *et al.*, 2003). Another US study reviewed 78 GP consultations concerning HIV risk and found that in most of the interviews the doctor avoided the discussion of HIV by changing the topic, not pursuing patient cues, or ignoring a stated concern (Epstein *et al.*, 1998).

In the previous chapter, the point was made that when you are a part of the mainstream culture, it is easy to be blind to the fact that you have any cultural baggage at all and to think that culture is something that only *other* people have. The next step is to measure how different those other cultures are from what you unthinkingly regard as 'normal'. A similar point could be made about sexuality. If you are part of the mainstream heterosexual (straight) culture, then it is easy to be blind to the fact that you also have a sexuality. Without reflecting on it, you might unconsciously measure anyone else's sexuality in relation to your own ideas of what is 'normal', without appreciating that we are all carrying around our own baggage about sex and sexuality, just as we are all carrying our own cultural baggage. The point that comes across quite strongly from the research evidence is that, as well the patient's own religious and moral framework, and level of comfort with discussing the subject of sex, it is just as often the doctor's own attitudes to sex and sexuality that they bring to discussions about sex with patients that influence whether or not the topic is handled well.

Talking about sex with older people

One other factor that many medical students and younger doctors can find difficult is the difference in age between themselves and their patients. It can be problematical to talk about sex to patients, particularly those of the opposite gender, who may be as old as your parents or grandparents. This discomfort in discussing

sex between doctor and patient across the generations can cut both ways of course. Sexual health is often thought of as only an issue for young people. However, while older people are unlikely to need contraceptive or pregnancy advice, and transmission of sexually transmitted infections is most common among people in their 20s, some sexual health problems, such as erectile dysfunction, vaginal dryness, or loss of libido, may be more common in older people (Gott *et al.*, 2004).

Doctors are often worried that they may cause offence by raising the issue of sex with older patients, despite the fact that there is little evidence of offence being inadvertently caused when they do. For example, a UK study of 22 GPs found that doctors found talking about sex to older people difficult, as it was not a topic they would normally discuss with people of this age group, and they did not see it as a 'legitimate' topic for discussion with them. Many of the doctors' beliefs were based on stereotyped views of ageing and sexuality, and they rarely initiated discussions about sexual health with older patients, although they acknowledged that older people themselves experienced difficulty in initiating such discussions and rarely did so (Gott *et al.*, 2004).

Talking with lesbian, gay, bisexual, and transgender patients

As well as not meeting the sexual health needs of older patients, another area where the medical profession has a poor record is in dealing with the needs of lesbian, gay, bisexual, and transgender (LGBT) patients. Although for obvious reasons it is difficult to quantify precisely, surveys indicate that probably around 3% of people are LGBT (Johnson *et al.*, 2001).

The consequences of homophobia

There have undoubtedly been enormous cultural shifts in most Western societies' attitudes to LGBT people in the past 40 years, and much progress has been made in fighting discrimination. Calls for the 'de-medicalization' of homosexuality echo the calls made by disabled people for the de-medicalization of disability. (See Smith *et al.*, 2004, for a discussion of barbaric medical 'treatments' used up until the 1970s to 'cure' homosexuality.) Homosexuality was included in the Diagnostic and Statistical Manual of Mental Disorders until 1973 (Rose, 1994) and astonishingly was only removed from the International Classification of Diseases, 10th revision (ICD-10) in 1992.

Despite the softening of attitudes in some places, homophobia (fear, hatred, or more generally discrimination against LGBT people) still persists. For example, one UK survey of 1285 gay and bisexual men and women found that 83% reported having experienced discrimination, either damage to property, personal attacks, or verbal insults, or insults or bullying at school, and 66% of those attributed this discrimination to their sexuality. There was also a strong statistical relationship between experience of discrimination and thoughts of suicide, as well as high rates of planned and actual deliberate self-harm, and high levels of mental illness among gay men (42%), lesbians (43%), and bisexual men and women (49%). These figures are high when compared with surveys of predominantly heterosexual people, where reported prevalence rates of mental disorder were 20% in women and 12% in men (Warner *et al.*, 2004). Other studies have shown that both lesbians and gay men avoid routine healthcare, prevention, and treatment services, attributed to fear of the consequences of disclosing their sexual identity because of perceived insensitivity on behalf of healthcare professionals. LGBT patient dissatisfaction with healthcare is also high (Bonvicini & Perlin, 2003).

There is not (yet) a duty on public bodies under UK law requiring them to promote equality of service for gay people, as already exists for gender, ethnicity, and disability. However, since 2007 it has been unlawful in the UK to discriminate against LGBT people in the provision of goods and services, which includes the provision of healthcare, housing, and other public services. The UK General Medical Council views discrimination against LGBT people as grounds to question a doctor's fitness to practice (Hunt & Dick, 2008).

Doctors' discomfort in talking to LGBT patients

The research evidence suggests that homophobia still exists in the medical profession. Frequently doctors assume that their patients are heterosexual, making subsequent disclosure of their sexuality – 'coming out' – difficult for patients. For example, one study of 22 UK GPs' attitudes to talking with their LGBT patients found that for almost half of them this could form a barrier to talking about sexual health, with a minority expressing overtly homophobic views. The doctors' difficulties related primarily to ignorance about LGBT people, and some felt discomfort or distaste emanating from various beliefs, ranging from feelings about sexual acts to beliefs about the nature of LGBT relationships, including stereotyping gay men as promiscuous (Hinchliff *et al.*, 2005).

Another Swedish study of 76 GPs' awareness of lesbian-related health issues found that assumptions of heterosexuality kept lesbian patients invisible to the doctors. Only 11% of the doctors knew of any issues relevant to lesbians, and only 32% were aware of having had any lesbian patients, despite having many years of practice, and no doubt having had many hundreds of lesbian patients among the thousands of patients they would have seen over the years. Only 5% had ever asked their patients about their sexual identity, and most questions concerning the patients' social network were framed in terms of the heterosexual nuclear family, for example, **'Are you married or single?'**, or **'How is your relationship with your husband?'** The GPs felt that it was up to the patient to mention it if they were a lesbian, unless the presenting issue was related to psychiatric, gynaecological, or psychosocial disease (Westerstahl *et al.*, 2002).

HOW TO OFFER A MESSAGE OF ACCEPTANCE AND INCLUSION OF LGBT PATIENTS AND COLLEAGUES

- Until you know a person's sexual identity, use gender-neutral and sensitive language, such as: **'Do you have a partner?'** or, **'Are you currently in a relationship?'** rather than, **'Are you married?'**, and **'Do you need to discuss contraception?'** rather than, **'What type of contraception are you using?'**

- Let patients provide information at their own pace with encouraging statements: **'I'm happy to discuss any concerns you have.'**

- Explain why such personal details need to be asked; for example, **'It would be helpful for me to understand this so that I can make an accurate assessment of your health needs.'**

- Ask the patient about any aspect of their lives that is unfamiliar to you.

- Role-model sensitivity and non-discrimination to colleagues and staff.

Bonvicini & Perlin (2003)

The experience of LGBT medical students and doctors

The assumption of heterosexuality applies not only to patients, but also to colleagues within the medical profession. For example, one UK study of 20 gay and eight heterosexual doctors found that most of the heterosexual doctors assumed that their colleagues were heterosexual and consequently were unaware of the effects that their remarks might have on their gay colleagues. Many of the interviewees reported anti-gay remarks being made by colleagues in front of gay medical students and doctors. For the gay doctors, anti-gay prejudice caused them extra stress, and they feared coming out because of the effect on their job prospects (Rose, 1994). Similarly, another more recent Canadian study of 29 gay and lesbian medical students found that they expended considerable energy assessing the safety of their training environments and trying to balance self-protection and self-disclosure. The students also had concerns that disclosing their sexuality would harm their career or lead to negative assessments (Risdon *et al.*, 2000).

When you might need to talk about sex in more detail

Some students are unclear about the appropriateness of asking personal questions about sex and relationships to all patients. In the course of a standard medical history, you should ask all patients if they have any sexual or relationship issues they want to discuss. You will need to use your judgement about when to ask more detailed questions about sex. If a patient presents with the common cold, you don't need to ask them if they masturbate! However, if their problem is erectile dysfunction, then it *is* appropriate to take a more detailed sexual history, including asking about masturbation.

Approach the subject by using a neutral open question like, **'Do you have a partner?'** or, **'Are you in a relationship at the moment?'** or, **'Are you currently sexual active?'** followed by, **'And how is your relationship?'** This will allow a patient who wants to talk further to expand, without them having to raise the subject themselves. By asking about sex in a sensitive way, you are signalling to the patient that, if they want to talk about sexual matters, then you are open to listen. If a patient does not want to talk about it, they won't, and provided the question has been phrased in a non-intrusive way, you do not need to worry that you will seem to be prying or will offend them. If, on the other hand, the patient wants to talk about their sexual problems, then you are giving them permission and an opportunity to do so.

Patients may introduce their real agenda tentatively, either in a consultation ostensibly about some other problem (**'And by the way . . .'**) or by using euphemisms or vague language. Their body language can provide a clue – they may look uncomfortable, or nervous, or

be defensive or blush. In this context, just because a patient looks uncomfortable with the topic, it does not mean that they don't want to talk about it. Ask them, **'Is there something else you'd like to discuss with me?'** Remember that patients may feel ashamed or even humiliated talking about their sexual problems. Patients need to feel that they can talk openly and frankly with you, that you will not be shocked by anything they tell you, and that you will not judge them. Try to be as matter of fact as possible, don't look embarrassed, and remember to stress the confidential nature of the discussion.

One of the difficulties in discussing sex relates to the choice of which words to use. You cannot assume that every patient will understand 'medical' words like masturbation, penis, vagina, fellatio, and so on. On the other hand, words that for many lay people are everyday language – 'fuck' for example – would be inappropriate for a health professional to use. Although patients may use crude language themselves, they are unlikely to expect their doctor to reflect that language back to them, even if the doctor is comfortable with it, which they may not be. If a patient says, **'It hurts when I'm fucking . . .'**, then when you summarize or reflect this back to them, you can say, **'Okay, so you said it hurts when you have sex. Can you tell me more about that?'** This sends a pretty strong signal that **'having sex'** is a phrase you are comfortable with. A similar strategy can be used for other sexual slang.

> ### QUESTIONS TO BE ASKED IN A SEXUAL HISTORY
> - What is the problem as the patient sees it?
> - How long has the problem been present?
> - Is the problem related to time, place, or partner? For example, if the problem is erectile dysfunction, does the man get erections during the night or on waking?
> - Is there a loss of sex drive or dislike of sexual contact?
> - Are there problems in the relationship?
> - Are there stress factors, anxiety, guilt, or anger not expressed?
> - Are there physical problems such as pain felt by either patient or partner?
>
> **Tomlinson (1998)**

Components of a full sexual history

A sexual history needs to cover anything that may affect sexual desire, arousal, and performance. As well as exploring the presenting problem, and the medical signs and symptoms, you will need to explore in detail the patient's relationship history in order to put the sexual issue into context. You will need to ask whether they currently have a partner and if so for how long they have been together, and you will need to ask about their previous partners and sexual activities. For people in relationships, you should ask whether they have any children and whether there is any obvious source of stress in the relationship or from other causes, such as work or finances. You should also ask whether the partner needs to be involved, perhaps in a future joint meeting, and explore the patient's and their partner's ideas about the problem. For women, you will need to ask about their contraceptive history and any past pregnancies, miscarriages, or terminations of pregnancy (abortions). Remember to include information about alcohol intake, medications taken, and, if appropriate, any recreational drug use, such as cannabis, as well as other possibly relevant factors, such as travel. There may be relevant cultural or religious rules and practices to explore. Remain non-judgemental about sexual practices, but use the opportunity for health promotion if it is appropriate.

SOME TIPS AND GOOD PRACTICE GUIDELINES WHEN TALKING ABOUT SEX AND SEXUALITY

Be direct:

- 'Would it be okay if I asked you some personal questions about your sexual relationships?'

Use generalized statements to make patients feel that they are 'normal' and that you are not judging them. For example:

- 'Many men experience difficulties with getting an erection at some point in their lives.'

- 'It's not unusual for us to see people who have picked up a sexually transmitted infection when they have been travelling abroad.'

- 'One possible explanation for your symptoms is that they're caused by a sexually transmitted infection. Do you think that's a possibility?'

When you need to ask more specific questions, use simple and unambiguous language, and encourage the patient to elaborate on their statements. For example:

- 'When you have sex with your partner, what do you do . . . ? And as well as that, do you do anything else?'

- 'When you say you had sex, was this vaginal, oral, or anal sex?'

Notice that closed questions can be useful in this context, when an open question might exacerbate a patient's embarrassment.

Use language that both you and the patient are comfortable with and understand (see above) and clarify any words or expressions you do not understand. For example:

- 'I'm sorry but I don't know that expression. What do you mean by that?'

Try to avoid using 'ever' or 'always' – they suggest a 'correct' answer. For example:

- 'Do you use condoms? Is that every time you have sex?'

- 'Did you have anal sex?'

- 'Have you had sex with anyone other than your partner?'

Similarly, remember that patients are likely to respond to questions like 'How often do you have sex?' by giving the answer they think is 'normal'. Some people might think having sex 'often' means twice a day, others might interpret that as once a week or once a month.

If you're not sure about the gender of the partner, try asking:

- 'Tell me more about your partner . . .'

If the answer is still not clear, and you need to know, ask directly and do not apologize:

- 'I need to ask you, is your partner a man or a woman?'

Keep a 'poker face', try to be as matter of fact as possible and don't look shocked or embarrassed, even if you are.

Finally, and most importantly, be empathic and avoid passing moral judgements.

Summary

Sex and sexuality are issues not only when patients have a 'sexual health' problem. All sorts of medical and psychosocial problems can have an impact on a patient's ability to have and to enjoy sex. Try to avoid making assumptions based on stereotypical ideas you may have, for example, that older people do not have sex, or that every patient must be heterosexual unless they tell you otherwise. Remember to ask all patients about their partners and relationships, and give them 'permission' and space to tell you about their sexual relationships or difficulties if they want to.

Further reading

Visit the Online Resource Centre for *Clinical Communication Skills* at: www.oxfordtextbooks.co.uk/orc/washer

References

Bonvicini, K. and Perlin, M. (2003). The same but different: Clinician–patient communication with gay and lesbian patients. *Patient Education and Counselling*, **51**, 115–122.

Epstein, R.M., Morse, D.S., Frankel, R.M., Frarey, L., Anderson, K., and Beckman, H.B. (1998). Awkward moments in patient–physician communication about HIV risk. *Annals of Internal Medicine*, **128**(6), 435–42.

Fayers, T., Crowley, T., Jenkins, J., and Cahill, D. (2003). Medical student awareness of sexual health is poor. *International Journal of STD and AIDS*, **14**(6), 386–389.

Gott, M., Hinchliff, S., and Galena, E. (2004). General practitioner attitudes to discussing sexual health issues with older people. *Social Science and Medicine*, **58**(11), 2093–2103.

Hinchliff, S., Gott, M., and Galena, E. (2005). 'I daresay I might find it embarrassing': General practitioners' perspectives on discussing sexual health issues with lesbian and gay patients. *Health and Social Care in the Community*, **13**(4), 345–353.

Hunt, R. and Dick, S. (2008). *Serves You Right: Lesbian and Gay People's Expectations of Discrimination.* London: Stonewall.

Johnson, A., Mercer, C., Erens, B., Copas, A., MacManus, S., Wellings, K., Fenton, K., Korovessis, C., Macdowall, W., Nanchahai, K., Purdon, S., and Field, J. (2001). Sexual behaviour in Britain: Partnerships, practices, and HIV risk behaviours. *The Lancet*, **358**(1835), 1842.

McKelvey, R., Webb, J., Baldassar, L., Robinson, S., and Riley, G. (1999). Sex knowledge and sexual attitudes among medical and nursing students. *Australian and New Zealand Journal of Psychiatry*, **33**, 260–266.

Risdon, C., Cook, D., and Willms, D. (2000). Gay and lesbian physicians in training: A qualitative study. *Canadian Medical Association Journal*, **162**(3), 331–334.

Rose, L. (1994). Homophobia among doctors. *British Medical Journal*, **308**(6928), 586–587.

Smith, G., Bartlett, A., and King, M. (2004). Treatments of homosexuality in Britain since the 1950s – An oral history: The experience of patients. *British Medical Journal*, **328**(7437), 427.

Tomlinson, J. (1998). ABC of sexual health: Taking a sexual history. *British Medical Journal*, **317**(7172), 1573–1576.

Verhoeven, V., Bovijn, K., Helder, A., Peremans, L., Hermann, I., van Royen, P., Deenkens, J., and Avonts, D. (2003). Discussing STIs: Doctors are from Mars, patients from Venus. *Family Practice*, **20**(1), 11–15.

Warner, J., McKeown, E., Griffin, M., Johnson, K., Ramsay, A., Cort, C., and King, M. (2004). Rates and predictors of mental illness in gay men, lesbians and bisexual men and women: Results from a survey based in England and Wales. *The British Journal of Psychiatry*, **185**(6), 479–485.

Westerstahl, A., Segesten, K., and Bjorkelund, C. (2002). GPs and lesbian women in the consultation: Issues of awareness and knowledge. *Scandinavian Journal of Primary Health Care*, **20**(4), 203–207.

WHO (2002). *Sexual Health.* Geneva: The World Health Organization.

CHAPTER 10

Talking with children and young people

Caroline Fertleman and Peter Washer

Learning points

This chapter will:

◆ discuss some issues around talking with parents

◆ outline the different stages of child development and
give advice on how to talk with:
  ○ preschool children
  ○ school-age children
  ○ young people.

Talking with children can sometimes present difficulties for medical students for several reasons. Many
students may have had little, if any, experience with
children. Although there is now a trend to expand medical school entry to more mature students, still very
few medical students are themselves parents. Without
that experience, it can be difficult to identify with parents and with how parents feel when their child is ill.
This chapter will therefore begin by discussing parental
anxiety and how best to talk with worried parents. It
will then follow the development of children from
preschool age through to adolescence, and discuss the
different communication issues that arise for children
of different ages. Talking with very sick children is a
particularly challenging aspect of paediatric practice.
The subject of breaking bad news and of talking about
dying (with adults) are dealt with in Chapter 15 of this
book, although it is unlikely that anyone but a senior
doctor would have to break very bad news to a child or
to his or her parents. Therefore, this chapter will focus
on the communication skills that medical students and

junior doctors would be expected to demonstrate when talking with children, young people, and their parents.

Talking with parents

Elsewhere in this book, the importance of involving patients' families and social networks in their care has been emphasized. This is particularly true when caring for children, which in effect means caring for the whole family, including other siblings, who can feel marginalized by attention being focused on the sick child. Before adult or elderly hospitalized patients can be discharged, the healthcare team has to plan who is going to care for them at home. With children, however, the parents are usually the carers. Parents continue to care for their children alongside the nurses, doctors, and other professionals throughout the child's illness, whether in hospital or at home. It is also worth remembering that, however much experience and expertise a doctor may have with children, the parents are often far more knowledgeable about their particular child's condition than anyone else, and they will want to be actively involved in any decision-making process about their child's treatment.

Dealing with parental anxiety

Talking with parents can be more difficult than talking with other relatives. It is difficult to describe the level of anxiety that parents have for their children. From the outside, this can sometimes seem disproportionate compared with the symptoms the child has. It is common for parents to fear that their child is more seriously ill than he or she actually is. For example, one US study of 370 routine paediatric consultations found that in a third of the consultations the doctors felt that the level of concern was disproportionate to the presenting symptoms. Further questioning revealed that the parents actually had unspoken fears that something much more serious was wrong with their child than the ostensible reason for the visit. Those parents often had a family history of a serious life-threatening illness, or the child themselves had had a serious illness in the past, which the parent thought might be recurring. Often an authority figure, such as a grandparent or someone with a superior knowledge of illness such as a nurse, had raised doubt in the parents' minds and advised them to seek medical attention, or at any rate the parent thought the illness was going on too long or was a recurrent problem (Bass & Cohen, 1982). In these sorts of cases, it is always worth asking what prompted the parents to seek medical advice; the person behind the referral then often becomes apparent.

In most contexts, adults can make their own decisions about whether to have medical treatment and which treatments they will have. Parents have to make the decisions for their children around medical matters. These decisions will be based on their own experience of parenting, as well as messages from the wider culture, family, friends, and the media. Parents' decisions may not concur with medical advice, for example parents who do not want their children vaccinated, or at the other extreme, parents who want prescriptions for antibiotics for their children when that is not medically indicated. It is often difficult in these types of circumstances for doctors to explain why they are providing that advice or treatment while still maintaining the parents' trust and satisfaction. For example, one US study of 259 routine paediatric consultations found that 55% of parents interviewed before seeing the doctor expressed an expectation of a prescription for antibiotics for their children, although only 1% made a direct request for them. However, even without a direct request for antibiotics, doctors still picked up the parents' expectation in 34% of the consultations. Those parents who had expected their children would be prescribed antibiotics but who were not given them had a higher satisfaction score if they were told that they could receive antibiotics in future if the child's condition did not improve (Mangione-Smith *et al.*, 2001).

Talking with parents and children

Although very few medical students are (yet) parents themselves, we have all been children, and we all have memories of visiting the doctor, or perhaps visiting or being in hospital when we were children. As you approach the part of your course where you will be working with children, it is worth reflecting on those memories in order to put yourself in the mindset of a child, for whom a visit to the doctor's or to hospital can be a strange and often frightening experience.

The trend in Western societies is towards less authoritarian styles of parenting, and relationships between adults and children are increasingly characterized by a greater openness towards children (Tates & Meeuwesen, 2000) and to involve them in making decisions that affect their lives. These trends are reflected in the law, which in many countries now gives children the right to consent to, but not to refuse, medical treatment when they are of an age to understand the implications of the treatment being proposed.

Yet research suggests that children often still do not participate as actively as they might. For example, a Dutch study examined the 'turn-taking' patterns between doctors, parents, and children in 106 video-taped GP interviews over a 20-year period, and found that the children's contribution to the consultations was limited to about 9% of the time, compared with the GP's contribution of about 51%. Encouragingly, this study did find that, over the course of the 20 years studied, the children were increasingly participating more actively. During those interviews where the children were more excluded from the discussion, it was often the parent who was responsible for exclusion of the child. While carrying out the physical examination, the children were able to communicate directly with the doctor, who was then more likely to address the children while the parent had to step aside (Tates & Meeuwesen, 2000).

PODCAST

A parent's perspective

"The doctors talk to both of us. I notice they look at Sam and they look at me, but they tend to explain more to me. If he doesn't understand, on the way home he asks questions and I explain it to him afterwards. So he might not say, 'Doctor, I didn't understand.' He waits until we get home and then he would say to me, 'I didn't understand mum, can you tell me?' But the doctors try to explain. We are always together, and they always try to explain to both of us."

"And have you found it's changed over the time he has got older because he started having this condition when he was a baby and he's now nearly nine. Have you seen a change in the way . . . ?"

"I have, I have, because at the beginning the doctors always spoke to me, whereas now they look at my son, they ask him, and they check him."

Podcast – Debbie, mother of Sam, aged 8, who has thallassaemia

---

Elsewhere in this book, there are discussions of different types of three-way consultations, for example when talking with patients who do not speak English and need an interpreter. When talking with children and their parents, similar issues arise. In light of the research above, every effort should be made to include and involve the child as much as is appropriate to their age. It is important to make eye contact with all those present in the consultation. Even if the child is very young, they will be able to pick up on the body language and understand the negative and positive emotions

being communicated. Parents will find it reassuring if their child, however young, is included in the consultation. Parents of disabled children also find it helpful if their children are included in the consultation at an appropriate level. Clearly, a child's contribution to medical consultations will be related to their developmental stage, and they should be increasingly involved as they get older. You may wish to explain most of the management to the child first, and then when you feel you have reached their level of understanding you can explain the more detailed information to the parents. Often parents are used to being in charge and will take the lead unless you specifically encourage the child to be in control. It is important to allow the child to ask questions and to provide adequate time and space in the discussion for this to happen.

The next part of this chapter will examine the different communication issues that arise with children of different ages. Although children's maturity and understanding can vary widely, for convenience the following sections have been divided into preschool-age children, school-age children, and young people.

Talking with preschool-age children

Trying to talk with preschool-age children can sometimes be frustrating, particularly when they are crying because they are distressed, in pain, or frightened. Preschool children are incapable of seeing the world from another person's perspective and cannot understand that others might know more than they do. This is sometimes expressed as them not having developed a 'theory of mind' (Mitchell & Zeigler, 2007). At this age, they believe things happen to them because of their own actions, so they may perceive illness and hospitalization as a punishment for bad behaviour or happening as if by magic (Hart & Chesson, 1998). Children at this age also have a very simple and rigid understanding of the world – something is either good or bad. They may therefore believe that doctors and nurses who hurt them, for example by giving them injections or performing other painful procedures, have deliberately set out to harm them (Perry, 1994). At this age, they cannot understand that suffering now, for example enduring pain, will have a beneficial outcome for them later, for example going home sooner, because they have no sense of delayed gratification and a limited understanding of time.

Research indicates that previous experience can be important in how fearful children are when they encounter doctors and hospitals. One Australian study presented 15 healthy children of 3–5 years of age with a variety of medical equipment – band-aids, intravenous infusion bags, gloves, bandages, and so on. The children were observed at play with the equipment, and later interviewed to gauge their level of understanding of what it means to be sick, as well as what they knew about cancer, hospitals, and medical equipment. The researchers found that those children who had not previously been exposed to hospitals had a naïve, joyous curiosity, and unsophisticated understanding about the medical equipment. However, where the child had had even a secondary personal experience with hospitals, for example where a close relative had been ill or in hospital, they were less ready to play spontaneously with the equipment, and their understanding was characterized by more fearful descriptions (McGrath & Huff, 2001).

> ## TIPS FOR COMMUNICATING WITH PRESCHOOL-AGE CHILDREN
>
> ◆ Call the child by the name they are usually called.
>
> ◆ Get down to their level by bending at the knees rather than bending down and towering over them.
>
> ◆ Use simple language and familiar words.
>
> ◆ Talk with them at their pace – they may need information broken down and given in stages.
>
> ◆ Examine their toy or parent/carer first.
>
> ◆ Examine them on their parent's lap.
>
> ◆ Ask the parent's permission *and* explain to the child what you are proposing to do and seek their agreement. If you ask the child's permission to examine them first, they might say no!

Reading to small children can also help them to understand what is happening in terms of their illness. The charity *Action for Sick Children* provides a relevant book list. The link to their website is available via the Online Resource Centre for this book.

Talking with school-age children

As children mature, they gain a systematic progression in their understanding of ideas about illness. They gradually learn that there are germs that can make them ill, and later again they begin to understand the complexity of the mechanisms that interact to cause illness. One US study of 128 healthy children of various ages found that only at about 12–13 years of age did the children begin to understand that there are multiple

causes of illness, and that the body may respond variably to different factors that can cause or cure illness. Interviews with the children revealed that, although they might seem quite sophisticated when talking about other subjects, they often demonstrated less sophistication in their understanding of illness. Not until adolescence can a child be expected to associate a number of different symptoms into a unified illness or syndrome, and smaller children cannot be expected to understand, for example, the logic of taking medication by mouth for a rash on their skin (Perrin & Gerrity, 1981).

> ## TIPS FOR COMMUNICATING WITH SCHOOL-AGE CHILDREN
>
> ◆ Introduce yourself and ask them their name, age, and what school they attend, as these will be familiar topics for them.
>
> ◆ Explain why you are talking to them.
>
> ◆ Get them to sit between you and their parent so you divide your attention equally between communicating (talking and looking) with their parents.
>
> ◆ Ask them what is worrying them or why they have come to hospital.
>
> ◆ Find out what they call urine/faeces/genitals and use those words.
>
> ◆ Ask their parents for clarification if you do not understand them.
>
> ◆ Take time to introduce them to medical concepts, especially if they have a chronic condition. Children will be able to understand complex things if they are explained appropriately.
>
> ◆ Ask them about school and friendships – but remember that they may not be happy to answer this in front of their parents, especially if they are being bullied.
>
> ◆ Use words that they are likely to understand.
>
> ◆ Try to avoid speaking down to them – they will be less likely to cooperate.
>
> ◆ Speak at a pace that is right for them.
>
> ◆ Do not examine them if they are crying (even if you have seen doctors doing this). Instead, wait until they settle.
>
> ◆ Try to avoid making promises that you cannot keep, for example not to hurt them, as this will reduce their trust in you in the future.

All children need to play, and one of the best things about being a student working on a children's ward is that you will have the time and opportunity to play with the children. Clinical areas where young children are likely to spend time, such as accident and emergency departments and GPs' waiting rooms, should have toys and child-friendly resources for them. Children's wards often have dedicated play specialists, who incidentally you will find to be valuable resources of information about child development.

PODCAST

A patient's perspective

"Doctors are actually good because they talk, they understand, they understand my point of view, yeah that was just nice."

"Can you tell me more about what you thought was good about them?"

"If I needed to have injections they would do it on my count, like if I said can you do it on three and then I would count to three and then they'll do it."

"So one of the things that was really good from your point of view was that they would let you know if you were going to have treatment in advance so they wouldn't sort of surprise you with it. What about explaining things to you, were they any good at that?"

"They did explain a lot of these things to me. That's how I would like it. I liked to be kept in the loop, to know what was going on."

Podcast – Casey, aged 13, talking about his experience of having leukaemia

---

Talking with young people

Adolescence is a dynamic time of development, and the transition from child to young adult is marked by physical and psychological changes, as well as new social expectations and roles. Conflicts around these changes can produce challenging behaviour, particularly with regard to risk-taking such as smoking, drinking alcohol, and experimenting with illicit drugs (Christie & Viner, 2005). When the changes of adolescence coincide with illness, one way that young people express their rebellion may be through non-adherence to medical advice and treatment. A request from a doctor for cooperation with medical treatment can turn into another opportunity for them to assert their growing independence from adult control (Windebank & Spinetta, 2008).

PODCAST

A patient's perspective

"The only thing I would say that wasn't very good was when the doctors would prefer to talk to my mum, my parents, and wouldn't talk to me. I mean I was hard work, I admit that myself, I was very hard work, but I felt like they couldn't talk to me, they had to talk to my mum and I was the third party, you know? They'd tell my mum and then my mum would tell me, and I would tell my mum and she would tell the doctor. It just wasn't making a lot of sense to me. That is the only thing I could say that was quite bad about the whole thing."

"Right, so you would have preferred they had come directly to you . . . With your mum there or without your mum there?"

"Maybe with my mum there, but talk to both of us, because there were a few occasions when I was asked to leave the room so they could speak to my mum and I thought, I'm not a little kid, I'm 16, they should tell me what's going on."

Podcast – Megan, aged 17, talking about her experience of being in hospital

---

During this period, young people are also maturing sexually. Often sexual experimentation – and risk-taking – is another way that young people test the limits of authority as they negotiate their way into adulthood. When talking about issues relating to sex and sexuality with young people, research suggests that the qualities young people most respect and value, and which they are most likely to seek from health professionals, are:

- a positive attitude towards sex

- an awareness of and interest in the issues that concern young people

- a genuine interest in the young person's point of view.

Research also suggests that when health professionals talk with young people about sex, they should try to use the language and words that the young person uses, explain professional language, and use a mixture of professional and less formal, colloquial language (Aggleton, Oliver & Rivers, 1998).

TIPS FOR COMMUNICATING WITH YOUNG PEOPLE

- ◆ See them both with and without their parents.
- ◆ Respect their views.
- ◆ Stress confidentiality, but say that if you are worried about their safety you will have to report this upwards on a need-to-know basis.
- ◆ Ask about drugs, sex, alcohol, smoking, and their moods/depression (when you are alone with them).
- ◆ If appropriate, take a full adolescent psychosocial history using the HEAADSSS protocol (Christie & Viner, 2005) –
  - ◆ Home life
  - ◆ Education
  - ◆ Activities including sports
  - ◆ Affect
  - ◆ Drug use
  - ◆ Sex
  - ◆ Suicide, depression, and self-harm
  - ◆ Sleep
- ◆ Avoid patronizing them.
- ◆ Take their health concerns or worries seriously, however absurd they may seem.
- ◆ Try to avoid being shocked or judgemental about what they tell you.
- ◆ Be yourself and do not try to be 'cool'; for example, do not swear just because they do.

Summary

Although this chapter has emphasized many of the difficulties that can arise when working with children, it also needs to be said that children can be great fun to work with. Although parents can be difficult to deal with sometimes, their anxieties when their child is unwell are entirely natural, and should be expected and accommodated. Remember the importance of caring for the whole family, including other siblings who may feel excluded or neglected. All children mature slightly differently, and therefore children of the same age may have different communication needs. Assess the level of understanding of each child, and then pitch your questions and explanations to match, ensuring that both the parents and the child are involved in making decisions about their care.

Further reading

Mitchell P. and Ziegler F. (2007). *Fundamentals of Development: The Psychology of Childhood.* Hove: Psychology Press.

Visit the Online Resource Centre for *Clinical Communication Skills* at: www.oxfordtextbooks.co.uk/orc/washer

References

Aggleton, P., Oliver, C., and Rivers, K. (1998). *Reducing the Rate of Teenage Conceptions. The Implications of Research into Young People, Sex, Sexuality and Relationships.* London: The Health Education Authority.

Bass, L.W. and Cohen, R.L. (1982). Ostensible versus actual reasons for seeking pediatric attention: Another look at the parental ticket of admission. *Pediatrics*, **70**(6), 870–874.

Christie, D. and Viner, R. (2005). Adolescent development. *British Medical Journal*, **330**(7486), 301–304.

Hart, C. and Chesson, R. (1998). Children as consumers. *British Medical Journal*, **316**(7144), 1600–1603.

Mangione-Smith, R., McGlynn, E.A., Elliott, M.N., McDonald, L., Franz, C.E., and Kravitz, R.L. (2001). Parent expectations for antibiotics, physician–parent communication, and satisfaction. *Archives of Pediatric and Adolescent Medicine*, **155**(7), 800–806.

McGrath, P. and Huff, N. (2001). 'What is it?': Findings on preschoolers' responses to play with medical equipment. *Child: Care, Health and Development*, **27**(5), 451–462.

Mitchell, P. and Zeigler, F. (2007). *Fundamentals of Development: The Psychology of Childhood.* Hove: Psychology Press.

Perrin, E.C. and Gerrity, P.S. (1981). There's a demon in your belly: Children's understanding of illness. *Pediatrics*, **67**(6), 841–849.

Perry, J. (1994). Communicating with toddlers in hospital. *Paediatric Nursing*, **6**(5), 14–17.

Tates, K. and Meeuwesen, L. (2000). 'Let mum have her say': Turntaking in doctor–parent–child communication. *Patient Education and Counselling*, **40**(2), 151–162.

Windebank, K. and Spinetta, J. (2008). Do as I say or die: Compliance in adolescents with cancer. *Pediatric Blood Cancer*, **50**, 1099–1100.

CHAPTER 11

Talking with people with mental health problems

Simon Michaelson and Peter Washer

Learning points

This chapter will:

- discuss the general issues around talking with people with mental health problems
- suggest questions you can use when taking a psychiatric history and mental state examination
- give advice on how to talk to patients with common psychiatric symptoms and disorders
- discuss alcohol and drug use, and how to approach these issues.

Mental illness is very common, and you will encounter many people with mental health problems throughout your career in various settings, both psychiatric and general. For example, a recent UK government survey (Office of National Statistics, 2001) found that:

- 1 in 6 people had a common mental disorder such as depression, anxiety, or phobias
- 1 in 200 was assessed as probably having a psychotic disorder such as schizophrenia
- 1 in 4 adults was assessed as having a hazardous pattern of drinking
- a significant minority of adults were assessed as alcohol and/or drug dependent.

Most mild to moderate mental illness has always been treated in primary care settings, and psychiatry is increasingly characterized by shorter stays in hospital than used to be the case, and by more acute or severe mental illness being managed in the community (Davies, 1997). Many patients with physical illness will also have a mental disorder, and mental ill health is particularly common in areas such as accident and emergency departments, where patients present with self-harm, alcohol and substance misuse, acute psychosis, and many other psychiatric problems.

General issues when talking with people with a mental disorder

Fundamentally, the communication skills you need when talking with a patient with mental health problems are the same as you need in any branch of medicine. You will need to use all the basic communication skills outlined in the early chapters of this book – active listening, attention to your own and to the patient's body language, appropriate use of questioning styles, avoiding jargon, responding to and following up their verbal and non-verbal cues, demonstrating empathy, and so on. Similarly, those parts of this book discussing how to talk about sex and sexuality, talk with people with medically unexplained symptoms and with people with dementia, as well as how to explore cultural issues and break bad news, and so on, are also very relevant in the context of psychiatry. Your goal in psychiatry, as in other contexts, is to build a rapport with the patient by giving them time to talk, being warm, and really listening and empathizing. Listening is in itself therapeutic, and patients often report that talking to students is helpful.

YOUR OWN SAFETY

Although people with mental illness are often stereotyped as dangerous, it is unusual for psychiatric patients to become violent. As in non-psychiatric settings, patients can become disturbed and aggressive, so be aware of the possibility, in order to minimize the risk. (See also Chapter 13 on dealing with angry patients and relatives.) Make sure that a colleague or staff member knows where you and the patient are, and, crucially, make sure you always sit nearest the door and keep it unlocked. Look out for signs that might indicate that the patient is becoming agitated, for example a change in posture, louder or more forceful speech, if they become abusive, or if there is an inappropriate change in the topic of conversation, for example to violent or sexual content. Never ignore your gut feelings, and if you feel uncomfortable or if you are in any doubt about the situation, leave the room immediately. Remember, if in doubt, get out!

Successfully engaging with patients with a mental disorder requires a sensitive and flexible approach. It is essential to take time to put patients at their ease. Start with informal general questions and build up a rapport before asking more specific questions. Students often experience some difficulty in phrasing questions about mental disorders. Try to use natural, everyday language, for example when expressing empathy: **'That must have been tough'** or, **'I imagine that's been really difficult for you.'**

In general medicine, patients are generally forthcoming with their main symptoms, but their underlying concerns can remain hidden. In psychiatry, some patients may not initially volunteer information in either of these areas, so you need to be particularly alert to both non-verbal and verbal cues, as these are crucial in uncovering patients' symptoms, ideas, concerns, and expectations, and in reaching a correct diagnosis. Look out for and respond to non-verbal cues, by asking, for example, **'You seemed distracted just then. Was something bothering you?'** It may be that the patient is hearing voices. Also look out for and reflect incongruities, for example, **'I noticed that when you said the break up hadn't bothered you, you seemed on the verge of tears.'** Also, be alert to, explore, and clarify any verbal cues, for example, **'What do you mean by depression?'** When patients say they feel 'paranoid', they usually mean self-conscious.

Patients who are very unwell, such as in severe depression, can have difficulty concentrating and get tired easily, so you need to give them more time to respond. Managing an interview can be a problem if, for example, an anxious or manic patient is jumping from topic to topic. In these circumstances, try saying something like, **'That sounds very interesting, but could we come back to that later?'** When dealing with sensitive topics, introduce them as understandable so that the patient feels more comfortable disclosing information. For example, **'When people are under severe stress, it's not uncommon to seek relief in other ways, such as drinking more alcohol or taking drugs. Has that happened to you?'** This also indicates that you will not be judgemental if they do disclose information.

Questions you can use when taking a psychiatric history and mental state examination

How to take a full psychiatric history is covered in detail in psychiatric textbooks (see suggested further reading below). The following section contains some additional suggestions, particularly about how you might phrase questions. Effective psychiatric interviewing is really a combination of good basic history taking coupled with effective communication skills. The structure and process of questioning is the same as in any medical interview (see Chapter 2). Compared with general medicine, you do not have to do everything in one interview; for example, you might say, **'This is really important, but I don't think we can do it justice in one interview. Can we arrange a time to talk about this tomorrow?'** Also, it is not always appropriate to follow the conventional order of a history. For example, if a patient is particularly keen to talk about family difficulties, then you could cover that area as it arises.

Generally, it is more effective to follow up any cues that suggest psychotic or other important symptoms as they arise, rather than wait to ask them directly in the mental state examination, although this may also be necessary.

THE SUBHEADINGS OF A PSYCHIATRIC HISTORY

- Presenting complaint(s)
- History of presenting complaint(s)
- Past psychiatric history
- Past medical history
- Family history
- Personal history (including social circumstances)
- Forensic history
- Personality (including alcohol and substance misuse)

Remember to start with open questions and let the patient speak uninterrupted for a few minutes. When taking a psychiatric history, there may be much more to discover than what the patient mentions spontaneously; for example, a patient may have both an acute depressive illness *and* alcohol dependence. For diagnostic purposes, find out which group of symptoms came first, by asking, **'Can you remember whether you felt depressed before you started drinking heavily or was it the other way round?'** It can help to be curious, as apparently insignificant changes, such as a patient stopping watching television, could be a cue to hidden symptoms, for example a belief that the television is talking

about them. Some patients with mental disorders deny a psychotic symptom if they are asked too directly, so it is important to watch out for, and respond to, cues while taking the history.

Wherever possible ask patients for specific examples with prompts such as, **'Can you remember when it last happened?'** If symptoms have been present for a long time, compare how the patient is currently feeling with how they usually feel, for example **'When were you last your normal self?'** and **'How do you feel now compared with when you were last well?'** Asking patients to describe a typical day can elicit a lot of information in disorders such as alcohol or substance misuse, and eating disorders.

When asking about the person's past history of mental disorder, begin by asking, **'Have you ever seen a psychiatrist or had any mental health difficulties in the past?'** Anything significant that arises should be explored in more detail. Physical illnesses can have psychiatric complications, particularly depression. When asking about a person's family history, rather than asking, **'Is there any history'** [note the jargon] **'of mental illness in your family?'**, ask instead, **'As far as you know, has anyone in your family had to see a psychiatrist or had any psychiatric problems?'** Patients often mention that someone had a 'nervous breakdown', if so, explore this further.

A personal history of trauma, especially sexual abuse, either as a child or an adult, is often present in a range of psychiatric disorders, such as eating disorder, deliberate self-harm, depression, and even psychosis. Approach this sensitive area by asking, **'I'd like to ask you some other questions about your background that we ask everybody. Is that okay?'** When asking about forensic history, use a screening question such as, **'Have you ever been in trouble with the law?'** Remember that when you ask about a person's personality, there will be many aspects to explore. Questions you might ask include, **'How do you see yourself compared with others?'**, **'How would other people who know you describe you?'**, **'How do you generally get on with others?'**, and **'How do you cope with stress?'**

The mental state examination

A psychiatric history covers the development of a patient's symptoms, but the mental state examination (MSE) focuses on the present. You will learn how to do proper MSEs during your psychiatry placement, and again this is covered in more detail in textbooks (see Further Reading). Essentially, it consists of a number of parts, which are listed in the box.

MENTAL STATE EXAMINATION
◆ Appearance and behaviour
◆ Speech
◆ Mood
◆ Thought form
◆ Thought content, including overvalued ideas, delusions, and suicidal/homicidal ideas
◆ Abnormal perceptions (including hallucinations)
◆ Cognitive function
◆ Insight

The art of a good MSE includes creating a vivid picture of how the patient is right now. This helps in confirming a diagnosis. For example, on medical wards, acute delirium (delirium tremens or 'DTs') can be mistaken for a non-organic psychiatric illness. Characteristic features in the mental state include fluctuating levels of consciousness, and disorientation, as well as lability of mood, distractibility, vivid illusions, and particularly visual hallucinations.

Most of the items of the MSE can be gathered during the history taking. The MSE should be restricted to information about the current illness and to observations made during the interview. You should write down verbatim any important statements the patient makes, such as those illustrating thought disorder. The use of transition statements or signposting is particularly important. If a patient is abruptly asked whether they are hearing voices, they might respond, **'Do you think I'm crazy?'** One way to approach these topics, including psychosis or cognitive function, is to frame it with a preliminary statement such as: **'I need to ask you some questions. Some of these may seem a bit unusual, and they may or may not apply to you, but they're routine.'** Insight has a number of components and is assessed by asking patients questions such as, **'Do you feel you are ill?'** and **'Do you feel that the illness is physical or mental?'**, as well as their understanding of the need for treatment and whether they will recover.

Talking with patients with common psychiatric disorders

Patients with psychosis

Patients are often relieved to be able to talk about their psychotic symptoms, even if doctors are sometimes reluctant to engage with patients' concerns about their psychotic symptoms (McCabe *et al.*, 2002). When enquiring about psychosis, use screening questions to identify any cues that can be followed up, such as: **'Have you ever felt anything unusual has been going on?'**, **'Do things around you seem odd or different?'**, or, **'Do you ever feel that people are playing tricks or games?'**

Once any cues are followed up, more specific questions can be asked, for example, **'Do you ever feel that people are trying to harm you or hurt you?'** or, **'Do you ever feel that you are being watched or followed?'** You should not argue with a patient's delusion, but at the same time you should not agree with them. Allow them to talk fully and openly about their abnormal beliefs and empathize with them by acknowledging the distress these ideas must cause. For example, **'I imagine it must feel awful to have those experiences'** or, **'You must be feeling pretty frightened by that.'**

Questions to ask people with psychosis (and what they screen for)

◆ **'Have you ever felt as if you were receiving messages from television, radio, newspapers?'** – ideas of reference

◆ **'Do you ever feel that your thoughts are being interfered with?'** – thought interference

◆ **'Do you ever feel that people can read your mind or that your thoughts are available to others?'** – thought broadcasting

◆ **'Have you ever felt as if thoughts are being taken out of your head?'** – thought withdrawal

◆ **'Do you ever feel that people are putting thoughts into your head?'** – thought insertion

◆ **'Do you ever feel that you are being controlled in some way, like a puppet?'** – passivity

It can be easy to mistakenly assume that thought interference and passivity are present. For example:

'Do you ever feel that you are being controlled?'

'It's the Government.'

but if explored further:

'How do you mean the Government is controlling you?'

'Well, you can't do anything these days without them passing laws; you can't even smoke in a pub anymore.'

It is important to assess the strength of a patient's conviction to assess whether it is a fixed delusion or an overvalued idea. Useful questions include:

- 'Are you absolutely sure that x is true, or is it possible that you might be mistaken?'
- 'If somebody else said that to you, what would you make of it?'

When patients say they are hearing voices

There are a number of important characteristics of voices that need to be elicited. Some patients will not spontaneously report hearing voices, but may describe people talking about them, which should be explored.

A screening question could be:

- 'Do you ever hear noises or voices that seem to come from nowhere or when there is no one around?'

If yes:

- 'Can you tell me more about what you hear?'

More specific questions include:

- 'What do they say?'
- 'Is there one voice or more than one voice?'
- 'Do you recognize the voices?'
- 'Do they seem to talk to you, like I'm talking to you, or about you, as if you're not there?' – second or third person
- 'Where do they seem to be coming from?'
- 'Do they seem to come from inside or outside your head?' – pseudohallucinations versus hallucinations
- 'Are they real or do you feel they are part of you?' – hallucinations versus pseudohallucinations
- 'How much of the time are they there?'
- 'Do you hear them in certain situations?'
- 'How do they affect you?'
- 'Do you ever hear your own thoughts spoken aloud?' – thought echo
- 'Do the voices ever tell you to do things?' – commanding voice

If yes, then ask:

- 'What do they instruct you to do?'
- 'Do they ever tell you to do bad things, for example hurt yourself or others?'
- 'Do you feel you have to act on them?'

Talking with depressed patients

If a patient mentions feeling depressed, then the severity and pattern of their depression, including frequency

and duration, should be explored in order to distinguish between normal sadness and a clinically significant depressed mood. Bear in mind that depressive illness can commonly just present with somatic symptoms or marked anxiety. The two central symptoms in making a diagnosis of clinical depression are a marked and persistent depressed mood and/or a pervasive lack of interest in usual activities. A commonly asked question, 'What is your interest like?' can confuse patients. A better alternative is, 'How much are you able to enjoy things compared with how you used to do?'

Specific biological symptoms of clinical depression need to be explored, including sleep and appetite. It is better to try and weave the questions into a natural dialogue, rather than ask a series of closed questions one after the other, which often causes patients to give briefer responses.

Examples of closed questions are:

'Do you sleep okay?' – closed/leading question

'Not really.'

'Do you have trouble getting off to sleep?'

'Yes, it takes me a while.'

'How long?'

'About an hour or two.'

The following is more efficient:

'It sounds like you've been feeling really quite depressed for some time. Has the depression affected you in other ways?'

'Yes, my sleep's terrible.'

'Could you tell me what happens when you go to bed at night?'

'Well, it can take me an hour or two to get off and then I keep waking up every hour or so.'

Assessing suicide risk

The risk of suicide should be assessed for all patients with depression and with any other serious mental disorder. You should not be afraid to ask about suicide directly; there used to be a myth that asking could implant an idea that might not have been there previously. In fact, if a patient is feeling suicidal, they usually welcome the opportunity to talk about it. It is common to enquire too bluntly, for example, 'Do you want to kill yourself?' A better approach is to ask a graded series of questions. This sensitive area can be introduced with a 'normalizing' statement, such as, 'These are routine questions we ask everybody.' This can then be linked to how they have been feeling, for example, **'Given how depressed you've felt recently, have you felt so bad that you thought life wasn't worth living?'**

The following questions should form part of a flowing dialogue:

- **'How do you see the future?'**
- **'Do you feel hopeless?'**
- **'Do you ever feel as if you don't want to carry on?'**
- **'Do you sometimes feel like you don't want to wake up in the morning?'**

If yes, then ask:

- **'Can you tell me more about these feelings?'**
- **'Have you ever had thoughts of harming yourself?'**

If a patient has had specific thoughts, ask:

- **'What particular thoughts went through your mind?'**
- **'Have you made any plans?'**
- **'How close have you come?'**
- **'What has stopped you doing anything?'**
- **'Have you actually tried to harm yourself?'**

If yes, then ask:

- **'What happened exactly?'**

If a patient has harmed themselves, this needs to be comprehensively assessed. Important areas to explore include what the person's intent was at the time, and how they feel afterwards, for instance are they happy they survived or do they wish they had succeeded.

Assessing risk to others

The potential risk that a patient may pose to others is not static, but can change over time. Pointers to higher risk include sociopathic personality disorder, alcohol and substance misuse, psychosis, and particularly any combination of these. Especially important are any threats the patient has made, any indecent acts carried out, and if they hear commanding voices or have persecutory delusions and morbid jealousy. The best predictor of the risk of future violence is a previous history of violence. Any aggressive act needs to be explored and documented thoroughly. Areas to cover include asking about what makes them angry, and whether they feel there is anyone in particular to blame for their problems.

Talking with anxious patients

Anxiety symptoms, especially panic attacks, can occur in many psychiatric disorders, either as primary or secondary symptoms. Anxiety and depression commonly coexist, and anxiety can often be the presenting symptom of depression.

You can ask:

- **'Do you ever get sudden bouts of anxiety?'**
- **'Could you describe a typical panic attack?'**
- **'When you get the panics, do you ever feel that something awful is about to happen to you?'**

Enquire about somatic anxiety symptoms, for example sweating and dizziness, as these can cause 'catastrophic' negative thoughts that fuel further panic attacks. For example:

- **'When you panic and experience the chest pain, do you ever feel like something bad is going to happen to you, like a heart attack?'**

You should also ask about avoidance. For example:

- **'Has the anxiety stopped you doing things you normally do?'**

In post-traumatic stress disorder, patients commonly experience nightmares and flashbacks, which can be elicited by asking, for example:

- **'Do you re-experience the accident?'**
- **'Do you ever get very vivid images of the (attack/ incident) as if you were almost back there?'**

Obsessional symptoms are thoughts, images, and actions that the patient feels compelled to repeat. These symptoms may be part of a primary obsessive compulsive disorder or secondary to another illness, especially depression, schizophrenia, or an organic disorder. These can be explored by asking:

- **'Do you ever find that you have to think certain thoughts or do certain things over and over again?'** – obsessional thoughts and compulsive rituals
- **'Do you find that you are checking a lot?'**
- **'Do you wash your hands over and over again?'**
- **'If you try and resist these thoughts (or rituals), do you worry something bad might happen?'**

Any symptoms should be explored in great (but not obsessional!) detail.

Assessing alcohol and drug use

Alcohol and drug misuse is prevalent in all Western societies, and when talking to patients you should always be alert for any cues, for example repeated mentions of drinking or a family history of alcohol or substance abuse. Within psychiatry, alcohol and drug use may be primary, or may be secondary to depression or social anxiety. The coexistence of substance misuse and psychosis is now exceedingly common.

Screening for alcohol problems

All patients should be asked how much alcohol they drink as part of a standard medical history. If a patient indicates that they are drinking above recommended levels (see Chapter 3), then they should be asked further questions to explore if their drinking is problematic. A useful question is to ask the patient to describe a typical day. The most widely used alcohol screening tool in clinical practice is the CAGE questionnaire, which identifies dependent rather than hazardous drinking patterns (Alcohol Concern, 2001). Symptoms of alcohol dependence syndrome should then be enquired about, including withdrawal symptoms and tolerance.

CAGE

C Have you ever felt that you should Cut down on your drinking?

A Have people Annoyed you by criticizing your drinking?

G Have you ever felt bad or Guilty about your drinking?

E Have you ever had a drink first thing in the morning, an 'Eye opener', to steady your nerves or get rid of a hangover?

Two positive responses are considered a positive result and indicate that further assessment is warranted (Alcohol Concern, 2001).

Talking with drug users

Drug users are often treated very badly by healthcare professionals, something that students soon pick up as part of the 'hidden curriculum'. For example, while those patients dependent on alcohol would routinely be provided with medication to prevent the symptoms of withdrawal, it is quite common for drug users' reports of symptoms to be disbelieved, and treatment for withdrawal symptoms withheld. It is very easy to sound judgemental and/or for patients to get defensive when discussing drug use. Try and be aware of your own feelings during an assessment. As well as a detailed history of the drug user, do not forget to include the impact on the user's life and on others

around him, as well as motivation to change by asking questions such as, **'Can you take me through a typical day?'** and **'What problems has it caused you?'**

STREET NAMES OF DRUGS

Street slang for drugs can be useful to know when you are talking to patients about their drug use, especially in accident and emergency departments.

amphetamine sulphate	speed, whizz
cannabis	marihuana (marijuana), draw, blow, black (for resin form), weed (for plant form), skunk (strong variety of plant form, often home grown)
cocaine (hydrochloride)	charlie, coke (powdered form)
crack	a shorter-acting but more powerful and more addictive form of cocaine
diamorphine	heroin, brown, smack, horse
lysergic acid diethylamide	LSD, acid, trips
methylenedioxy-methylamphetamine	MDMA, ecstasy, E
D-methamphetamine	crystal meth, ice, tina

Summary

As this chapter has indicated, although you will learn most of your psychiatry in your psychiatric placement, you will often encounter patients with mental disorders throughout your clinical training. The key to successful psychiatric interviewing involves allowing the patient to tell their story while flexibly using good communication skills and history taking, as well as being interested, sensitive, and showing empathy.

Further reading

Aquilina, C. and Warner, J. (2004). *A Guide to Psychiatric Examination*. Knutsford UK: Pastest.

Lewis, S. and Guthrie, E. (2002). *Master Medicine: Psychiatry: A Clinical Core Text with Self Assessment*. Oxford: Churchill Livingstone.

Stringer, S., Church, L., Davison, S., and Lipsedge, M. (Eds) (2009). *Psychiatry PRN – Principles, Reality, Next Steps*. Oxford: Oxford University Press.

Visit the Online Resource Centre for *Clinical Communication Skills* at: www.oxfordtextbooks.co.uk/orc/washer

References

Alcohol Concern (2001). *Screening Tools for Healthcare Settings*. London: Primary Care Alcohol Information Service.

Davies, T. (1997). ABC of mental health: Mental health assessment. *British Medical Journal*, **314**(7093), 1536–1539.

McCabe, R., Heath, C., Burns, T., and Priebe, S. (2002). Engagement of patients with psychosis in the consultation: Conversation analytic study. *British Medical Journal*, **325**(7373), 1148–1151.

Office of National Statistics (2001). *Psychiatric Morbidity Among Adults Living in Private Households*. London: HMSO.

CHAPTER 12

Giving information and managing uncertainty

Peter Washer

Learning points

This chapter will:

♦ describe best practice in explaining medical information

♦ discuss what to say when you don't know the answer

♦ describe different types of medical uncertainties and how to discuss these with patients

♦ discuss some of the issues around complementary and alternative medicine.

Taking a medical history, where you gather information and explore the patient's agenda, is given a great deal of prominence in medical education. However, the second part of the medical interview, where doctors give information, explain diagnoses and treatments, make decisions, and agree future management, is arguably neglected (Elwyn *et al.*, 1999b). As a result, research suggests that doctors may be less proficient in the skills required for giving information. For example, one Danish study contrasted simulated patient interviews between 22 students in the last semester of medical school and 23 experienced senior registrars with little or no training in communication. They found that both groups were lacking skills in terms of giving information, and both groups informed patients in a doctor-centred fashion with little regard for the patient's understanding, views, and emotions (Aspegren & Lonberg-Masden, 2005).

Perhaps one of the reasons for this emphasis on information gathering rather than giving is that, as a medical student, giving information is something that you are not permitted to do. As a medical student, you are (rightly) told that you are to refer patients who ask for information to a qualified health professional. However, you will find that the phrase **'I'm sorry but I'm *only* a medical student'** has a limited shelf life. When the transition to being a doctor does happen, you will be expected to explain diagnoses, prognoses, and treatments to patients, to answer their questions, and to check that they have understood what you have told them. The first part of this chapter will therefore describe ways of explaining medical information to patients, and subsequent chapters will describe ways of talking about medical errors, risk, and breaking bad news, and also deal with information giving in specific contexts.

PODCAST

A professional perspective

"Three and a half years ago you made this transition from being a medical student to being a doctor. I mean, how was that transition?"

"It was a really hard transition. I think that you're just not prepared for the idea. When you're a medical student you're now much more part of a team but when you are a doctor suddenly you're the person that has to make decisions, deal with the relatives, and not just the actors and people like that."

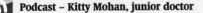 **Podcast – Kitty Mohan, junior doctor**

Another difficulty in the transition from medical student to doctor relates to how to manage uncertainty. The second part of this chapter will discuss different types of medical uncertainty, such as patients whose symptoms cannot be explained medically and patients who use alternative medicine, and will give some advice on how to talk about these uncertainties with your patients.

How to explain medical information

Although it has been said many times in this book in different contexts, probably the single most important thing to remember when you are giving patients information is to avoid medical jargon and to translate every term and concept from 'medspeak' into language pitched at a level that this particular patient is likely to understand.

PODCAST

A relative's perspective

"When you say you've had a problem understanding what the doctors were saying, what exactly do you mean?"

"Well, basically because they use their own jargon most of the time, this really for an everyday person it means nothing."

"So if the doctors were to use some sort of medical jargon or a medical concept you didn't understand, would you not just feel able to ask them to explain it to you?"

"Yes, of course I would. Sometimes I try to work it out in my head and try to make sense of what they are saying, thinking that I may be able to understand at the end of it what they were actually saying. But some other times they may use very technical terms, terms I really wouldn't understand, and if I repeat it, if I ask them to repeat it, they may repeat the same thing."

 Podcast – Alice, carer for her partner

Sometimes you will know in advance of meeting a patient that you have information to give them, for example if you are giving the results of a test. If you have the opportunity, make a mental plan of what you are going to say beforehand. Consider how you are going to phrase the information and translate any jargon. Think what your responses will be to the more obvious questions they are likely to ask, for example: **'Will it hurt?'**, **'Will I recover completely?'**, **'Will I be left with a scar?'** In particular, think of the information you do not have or cannot be certain about and how you are going to deal with that (see below).

In most cases, before you give information or explanations you should start by asking the patient to tell you what they understand so far, and if appropriate what they expect from the consultation. There might be exceptional cases where you can 'cut to the chase' a little quicker; for example, if a patient has come for the result of a test, they will be anxious and probably will not appreciate a long preamble. In these cases, you can open the interview by saying, **'You had a test for x last**

week; we have the results back and . . .' (followed by a warning shot if it is bad news).

It sometimes helps for you to signpost the structure of the consultation at the outset. Tell the patient that you are going to explain what the problem is, and that then you are going to explain the options regarding what can be done to help. You can also encourage the patient to stop you and ask any questions that arise at any point. Remember though, that you will still need to stop at the end of each section to check that they have understood, and to ask them if they have any questions at that point before you move on. This is sometimes called 'chunking and checking', that is, giving information in small chunks and then checking it has been understood by summarizing, and asking if the patient has any questions *before* you move on to the next section. Don't forget, some people understand visual or written information more readily – use drawings and diagrams, and give any other forms of patient information such as leaflets if you have them.

Remember that people do not listen well when they are distressed or anxious. Repeat phrases gently and ask them if they wish to continue. Watch closely for any cues that they are giving you and respond to those cues. If they look upset, think about how much detail they need at this stage. It might not be effective, safe, or kind to try to cover everything in one interview, so you might need to arrange a follow-up appointment to continue the discussion. Also, think about social support – do they have someone at home to talk this through with? Ask, **'Who's at home with you?'**, **'Would you like to come back with someone to support you and we can discuss the next stage together?'** and if so **'Would you like me to explain this to your family/partner, or do you want to talk to them yourself first?'**

Remember that patients will forget to ask things that are important, forget bits of information they have been told, and think of new issues to ask about after the consultation is over. Tell them, **'I'm sure you'll think of a million questions you'll want to ask me later – write them down, and we can deal with them when we next meet.'**

At the end of the consultation, check for understanding by repeating and clarifying. Summarize the main points – think of this as a verbal bullet point list. Finally, check whether there is anything at all they would like to ask at this stage. Always end by saying what happens next – usually the next appointment, but it might be that they have to go back to the waiting room and wait for a nurse to call them and so on. When appropriate, consider how they are getting home and whether they need transport organized for them. Give them your contact details if necessary and appropriate.

The Calgary–Cambridge guide, which was discussed in Chapter 3, also has a structured list that you may find useful when giving information. A link to this guide is available via the Online Resource Centre associated with this book.

What to say when you don't know the answer

Often medical students think that patients and relatives are asking for detailed medical information when in fact the person is only looking for general reassurance. It is possible to give reassurance without crossing the boundaries of what you are and are not allowed to say as a medical student. You should avoid empty or false reassurances, such as, **'I'm sure it'll be alright'**, even though that might be what the patient wants to hear, and indeed what you would like to be able to tell them. However, both as a medical student and as a doctor, you can be helpful without giving false reassurance. Here are some examples of reassurance you might use:

REASSURING PHRASES

'You did the right thing by . . . [going to the doctor/calling the ambulance, etc.] when you did.'

'You're in the right place.'

'There is a team of experts here/there who will be able to find out what's wrong and help you.'

'Everything possible will be done to help you . . .'

'I'm a medical student [not I'm only a medical student] and so I'm not the best person to be explaining things to you, but . . .'

'I can see you're concerned/worried/upset.'

'I'll make sure the doctor is aware of your concerns and will come and talk to you.'

'A doctor will see you as soon as possible.'

'Dr . . . is a really good doctor.'

'It's not possible to say at the moment what might be wrong – that's why we need to do more tests so that we can find out.'

'This will hurt, but the pain will pass quickly. If the pain gets too much then let me know and I'll stop until you're ready to continue.'

Different types of medical uncertainties

In an influential work about the socialization of medical students carried out at Cornell University medical school in the 1950s, and which is still resonant today, Fox (1957) identified three different origins of medical uncertainty:

- The first related to limitations of the students' own knowledge.

- The second related to limitations of medical knowledge.

- The third related to the challenge of distinguishing between these two.

She described how the approaches to uncertainty taken by students evolved throughout medical training; from an anxious focus on the students' own individual limitations of knowledge towards an acceptance and accommodation of limitations in the field, until they developed a doctor-like 'manner of certitude', realizing that it was important to act like a *savant* even when they did not actually feel that certain.

A more recent Canadian study expanded this framework by adding other sources of uncertainty, including (Lingard *et al.*, 2003):

- the limitations of evidence (for example to make a firm diagnosis)

- limitless possibility ('everything's possible')

- the limitations of the patient's account

- the limits of professional agreement (some doctors would do this, others would do that)

- the limitations of scientific knowledge (where no one really knows).

The rest of this chapter will examine these different aspects of medical uncertainty. In particular, it will examine the issues when patients present with symptoms that cannot be explained medically, and when patients seek alternatives to conventional medicine.

Patients often present with problems that are social or psychological rather than medical in origin, and thus do not have a clear set of signs and symptoms that add up to a certain diagnosis (Bligh, 1999). Whereas illness attributed to physical causes elicits concern and compassion, those attributed to psychosocial causes tend to be viewed as controllable and elicit less compassion, and may even evoke anger in doctors (Kirmayer *et al.*, 2004). For example, one Norwegian study surveyed 886 medical students and doctors, and asked them to rate different diseases on a scale of prestige. They found diseases associated with medically sophisticated, immediate, and invasive procedures were given high prestige, especially where they affected the young or middle-aged, and where they were thought to strike at random. High-prestige diseases included myocardial infarction, leukaemia, testicular cancer, and brain tumours. Diseases without so-called objective diagnostic signs were generally accorded a low prestige, as were those associated with an 'intemperate lifestyle'; these included cirrhosis of the liver, depression, schizophrenia, anorexia nervosa, and anxiety (Album & Westin, 2008).

Medically unexplained symptoms – 'somatization'

People who are under stress often react by drinking alcohol excessively, smoking cigarettes, or taking illicit drugs. Some people 'comfort eat' when they are unhappy. Other people react to stress by worrying about their health and feeling ill; in effect, expressing their psychosocial distress as physical symptoms. At one end of a spectrum are what are sometimes called the 'worried well'. This is a normal stress reaction, and the physical symptoms that these people complain of will go away when the things that stress them subside. The worried well often seek medical attention, but they are amenable to appropriate reassurance from a doctor. Indeed, many medical students suffer this type of stress reaction when they first have contact with very ill people and convince themselves they have a similar disease (Barsky, 1988).

At the other end of this spectrum of expressing psychosocial difficulties as physical symptoms are those people who have a psychiatric illness – somatization disorder – where their hypochondria becomes almost a way of life. They believe that they are gravely ill, that they have symptoms that cannot be explained medically, they are preoccupied with their health, and they have unhappy relationships with doctors (Barsky, 1988). The World Health Organization's International Classification of Diseases (ICD-10) defines somatization disorder as the '*repeated presentation of physical symptoms, together with persistent requests for medical investigations, in spite of repeated negative findings and reassurances by doctors that the symptoms have no physical basis*' (Rosendal *et al.*, 2005).

However, the word 'somatization' is often used in a looser sense, to refer not to a psychiatric illness, but as shorthand for unexplained medical symptoms (Gill &

Sharpe, 1999). These patients often present with vague and multiple symptoms such as tension headache, chronic fatigue, and unexplained chronic pain, which cannot be accounted for by a diagnosable physical disease. Of course, medically unexplained symptoms may have an organic cause that just has not *yet* been identified because the underlying disease is difficult to diagnose, for example syndromes such as systemic lupus erythematosus (Stockl, 2007). The prevalence of patients with medically unexplained symptoms is very high, particularly in general practice, where they make up an estimated 15–66% of all consultations (Epstein *et al.*, 1999; Kirmayer *et al.*, 2004; Kleinman *et al.*, 1978; Rosendal *et al.*, 2005).

Doctors often label these patients with blaming language, such as (for British doctors) 'difficult', or 'heartsink' patients, or (for US doctors) 'crocks', 'trolls', 'turkeys', or 'gomers' (standing for 'get out of my emergency room'). However, these labels describe the emotional reaction of the doctor rather than any common characteristic of the patients. This group of patients is perceived as aggressive and rude; they may demand certificates or doctors' letters, show little respect for the doctor's knowledge, set doctor against doctor, and generally cause disruption and distress (McDonald & O'Dowd, 1991). The dislike felt for these patients by doctors is often transmitted to other staff (O'Dowd, 1988), and medical students also soon learn this discourse as part of the 'hidden' medical curriculum. This may be an understandable defence mechanism for doctors, particularly GPs, who can feel helpless and frustrated when dealing with frequent attenders with endless complaints, the roots of which often lie in their unhappy lives, and which are not amenable to medical solutions.

From the perspective of doctors, the stereotypical 'heartsink' patient has little 'really' wrong with them, and they are often perceived as timewasters and malingerers. However, a systematic review of 34 studies principally from the UK, USA, and Scandinavia on frequent consulters found that these patients had multiple, complex problems. These problems included chronic physical disease, with or without social and psychiatric problems, although they did not see themselves as psychiatrically unwell. Women were over-represented, although this might reflect the generally higher consultation rates in women. Associations were found with single people, poverty, the unemployed, and those whose marriages had broken down. Patients who consulted more frequently were more likely to have a medical diagnosis and a less healthy lifestyle, and, in particular, problem drinking (Gill & Sharpe, 1999). The correlation between living alone and somatization is particularly telling. Contemporary Western societies are characterized by unstable family structures and a splintering of social relationships. For example, it was once common but is now rare for elderly parents to live with their married children. Without the feedback loops that come from living with others, the thought process goes something like: **'I'm feeling poorly today. Do I have chronic fatigue syndrome?'** In response to which there is no one there to reassure them, **'No, you're just sleeping poorly at the moment . . .'** (Shorter, 1992).

Talking with the somatizing patient

Patients experience *illness*, and the severity of their symptoms can be exacerbated by psychosocial stressors. Doctors diagnose *disease* when they can find an organic cause for the patient's illness. However, just as it is possible for disease to exist without illness or symptoms (in the early stages of cancer for example), it is also possible for illness to exist without there being underlying disease. These patients should be distinguished from malingerers, such as those patients who feign back pain to be signed off sick from work. The illness that the somatising patient describes is not imagined but is really experienced by them, and they understandably resist the moral blame that underlies the 'heartsink' label. One consequence is that they can become more vigorous in seeking healthcare and interventions. They often end up 'shopping' for doctors, or seeking alternative medicine (see below) (Epstein *et al.*, 1999). Patients and doctors alike share a medicalized culture that does not regard psychiatric illness as being as legitimate as 'proper' organic disease, and patients will thus refuse to accept the idea that they could be helped by psychotherapy and antidepressants, while often continuing on a fruitless quest for a medical disease diagnosis (Showalter, 1997).

What then are the best ways to move forward from this *impasse* of mutual blaming and hostility and to manage communication with these patients? Research suggests that:

♦ Patients with medically unexplained symptoms acknowledge and provide GPs with cues to their psychological needs. They seek emotional support rather than the disproportionate levels of somatic intervention they receive from doctors (Salmon *et al.*, 2005).

- Medical explanations that were perceived by patients as being consistent with the patient's essentially physical conception of the body and that involved them in an opportunity for self-management legitimized the patient's suffering, removed blame, and were experienced as satisfying and empowering (Salmon *et al.*, 1999).

- When the bodily quality and cultural meanings of their suffering are recognized, most patients will acknowledge that stress and emotions have an effect on their physical state. Focusing on the psychological and social factors that exacerbate symptoms may provide a rationale for behavioural medicine interventions that can improve adaptation (Kirmayer *et al.*, 2004).

- Doctors should try to build trust with these patients who may feel discounted and abandoned by other doctors. One strategy is to explore issues such as diet, physiotherapy, relaxation techniques, massage, and exercise. Provided they are not interpreted by the patient as discounting, these can contribute to non-specific healing that complements disease-specific treatment. Paradoxically, modest promises and objectives may result in greater patient satisfaction and health improvement (Epstein *et al.*, 1999).

Complementary and alternative medicine

Having medically unexplained symptoms does not always lead patients to try complementary and alternative medicine (CAM). Similarly, not all patients who use CAM do so because they have medically unexplained symptoms – CAM is widely used by patients with AIDS and cancer, for example. However, people often turn to CAM when they have exhausted every conventional medical option or because they are dissatisfied with what they see as inadequate explanatory frameworks for their illness. Indeed, many conventional doctors train and work in CAM, as they describe feeling alienated by 'objective' scientific medicine, which they see as fragmented and unsatisfying (Shohet, 2005). It seems appropriate, therefore, to discuss the issues that arise with alternative medicine here.

CAM is extremely popular around the world – around 50% of people in European countries such as France, Belgium, Germany, and Denmark, and around 70% of people in Australia, America, and Canada, have used CAM. A World Health Organization review found that the global market for CAM is worth over US$60 billion. In the UK, one in ten British people visit a CAM practitioner every year and the number of alternative practitioners in 2005 was estimated at 47,000 – more than the 35,000 British GPs (Shapiro, 2008).

The Western biomedical model looks to diagnose a *disease* from the patient's experience of *illness* – their signs and symptoms. This model is culturally specific, but, importantly, is shared by both doctors and patients, with an underlying assumption that organic disease is more 'real', significant, and interesting than illnesses that have psychosocial origins (Kleinman, Eisenberg & Good, 1978). By contrast, CAM practitioners base their treatments more on the way the patients experience and manifest their disease as opposed to directing treatment at underlying disease processes. They often provide explanations that make sense to patients, such as describing their illness in terms of environmental factors. Users of CAM cite increased opportunities for active participation in the process of recovery and the amount of time available for consultation as reasons for choosing CAM (1 hour for first appointments in comparison with the 7 minutes or so they typically get with a British GP) (Zollman & Vickers, 1999a).

THE EFFICACY OF CAM

Professor Edzard Ersnt is a medical doctor who in the past trained in and practised homeopathy, and is now Professor of Complementary Medicine at Exeter University. His book *Trick or Treatment*, written with the science writer Simon Singh, reviewed the results of hundreds of scientific papers on CAM. Their conclusions in relation to the four major strands of alternative medicine – acupuncture, homeopathy, chiropractic therapy, and herbal medicine – were:

'*While there is tentative evidence that acupuncture might be effective for some forms of pain relief and nausea, it fails to deliver any medical benefit in any other situation and its underlying concepts are meaningless. With respect to homeopathy, the evidence points to a bogus industry that offers patients nothing more than a fantasy. Chiropractors, on the other hand, might compete with physiotherapists in terms of treating some back problems, but all their other claims are beyond belief and carry a range of significant risks. Herbal medicine undoubtedly offers some interesting remedies, but they are significantly outnumbered by the unproven, disproven, and downright dangerous herbal medicines on the market.*'

Singh & Ernst (2008, p. 219)

Reasons why doctors may need to discuss CAM with patients

Even if the efficacy of many CAM therapies may be questionable in biomedical terms, it is important not to dismiss patients who seek advice regarding its use. The underlying motives of patients who are considering CAM may need exploring. For example, they may be experiencing unacceptable side effects from conventional medicines or have difficulties in adjusting to their illness. Rather than dismissing CAM on principle, doctors who listen and support their patients' choice, and whose advice minimizes risk, are more likely to warn patients off the more radical therapies (Tovey & Broom, 2007) and to encourage patients to use CAM appropriately, as an adjunct rather than an alternative to, conventional treatments (Zollman & Vickers, 1999b).

Another reason why it is important to keep channels of communication open regarding CAM is the potential for harmful interactions with conventional treatments. There is a widely held misconception that, because herbs are 'natural', they are entirely safe. Clearly, this is not the case – many plants are inherently poisonous. The most documented information on herb-drug interactions relates to St John's wort and warfarin (Fugh-Berman & Ernst, 2001), but St John's wort also interacts adversely with digoxin, theophylline, cyclosporin, HIV protease inhibitors, anticonvulsants, and oral contraceptives. Despite this, several studies report that CAM use is rarely documented in patients' notes (Cockayne, Duguid & Shenfield, 2004; Constable, Ham & Pirmohamed, 2006). Another consequence of the misconception that CAM therapies are natural and safe is that users may not associate adverse drug reactions with their use, or may be reluctant to report adverse reactions of herbal medicines to their GP or pharmacist (Barnes, 2003). Patients must be warned, therefore, about the risks of combining these products with conventional medicines (De Smet, 2006).

Useful questions when inquiring about the use of CAM are (from Zollman & Vickers, 1999b):

- Healthcare behaviour
  - 'Have you ever tried any other treatment approaches for this problem?'
  - 'Have you ever seen a complementary or alternative practitioner for this problem?'
  - 'Have you ever tried changing your diet because you thought it might help this problem?'
  - 'Have you used any herbal or natural remedies that you have bought from a chemist or health food shop?'

- Healthcare attitudes
  - 'What are you hoping will come out of your complementary treatment?'
  - 'What was it that encouraged you to try complementary medicine?'

- Communication and cooperation
  - 'Would you be prepared to ask your complementary therapist to let me know about your treatment and progress?'

Summary

The second half of a medical consultation is where patients are given information. As a medical student, you are not permitted to give information to patients, but this sometimes leaves students with the sense that, once qualified, you will suddenly have all the answers to patients' questions. One of the most difficult concepts to come to terms with as a medical student is that the practice of medicine is far more uncertain that it at first appears. As you mature into your new role, you will come to realize that patients' illnesses often will not have a neat medical solution. Your role as a doctor is as much to reassure and support people through their distress as it is to diagnose and treat their diseases. Acknowledge uncertainty, while at the same time stressing what you *do* know and what you *can* do to help.

Further reading

Visit the Online Resource Centre for *Clinical Communication Skills* at: www.oxfordtextbooks.co.uk/orc/washer

References

Album, D. and Westin, S. (2008). Do diseases have a prestige hierarchy? A survey among physicians and medical students. *Social Science and Medicine*, **66**, 182–188.

Aspegren, K. and Lonberg-Masden, P. (2005). Which basic communication skills in medicine are learnt spontaneously and which need to be taught and trained? *Medical Teacher*, **27**(6), 539–543.

Barnes, J. (2003). Quality, efficacy and safety of complementary medicines: Fashions, facts and the future. Part II: Efficacy and safety. *British Journal of Clinical Pharmacology*, **55**, 331–340.

Barsky, A.J. (1988). *Worried Sick: Our Troubled Quest for Wellness*. Boston and Toronto: Little, Brown and Company.

Bligh, J. (1999). Persistent attenders and heartsink. *Medical Education*, **33**(6), 398.

Cockayne, N., Duguid, M., and Shenfield, G. (2004). Health professionals rarely record history of complementary and alternative medicines. *British Journal of Clinical Pharmacology*, **59**(2), 254–258.

Constable, S., Ham, A., and Pirmohamed, M. (2006). Herbal medicines and acute medical emergency admissions to hospital. *British Journal of Clinical Pharmacology*, **63**(2), 247–248.

De Smet, P. (2006). Clinical risk management of herb–drug interactions. *British Journal of Clinical Pharmacology*, **63**(3), 258–267.

Elwyn, G., Edwards, A., and Kinnersley, P. (1999b). Shared decision-making in primary care: The neglected second half of the consultation. *British Journal of General Practice*, **49**(443), 477–482.

Epstein, R.M., Quill, T.E., and McWhinney, I.R. (1999). Somatization reconsidered: Incorporating the patient's experience of illness. *Archives of Internal Medicine*, **159**(3), 215–222.

Fox, R. (1957). Training for uncertainty. In: R. Merton, G. Reader, and P. Kendall (Eds), *The Student Physician: Introductory Studies in the Sociology of Medical Education*. Cambridge, Massachusetts: Harvard University Press.

Fugh-Berman, A. and Ernst, E. (2001). Herb–drug interactions: Review and assessment of report reliability. *British Journal of Clinical Pharmacology*, **52**, 587–595.

Gill, D. and Sharpe, M. (1999). Frequent consulters in general practice: A systematic review of studies of prevalence, associations and outcome. *Journal of Psychosomatic Research*, **47**(2), 115–130.

Kirmayer, L., Groleau, D., Looper, K., and Dao, M. (2004). Explaining medically unexplained symptoms. *Canadian Journal of Psychiatry*, **49**(10), 663–672.

Kleinman, A., Eisenberg, L., and Good, B. (1978). Culture, illness, and care: Clinical lessons from anthropologic and cross-cultural research. *Annals of Internal Medicine*, **88**(2), 251–258.

Lingard, L., Garwood, K., Schryer, C., and Spafford, M. (2003). A certain art of uncertainty: Case presentation and the development of professional identity. *Social Science & Medicine*, **56**(3), 603–616.

McDonald, P. and O'Dowd, T. (1991). The heartsink patient: A preliminary study. *Family Practice*, **8**, 112–116.

O'Dowd, T. (1988). Five years of heartsink patients in general practice. *British Medical Journal*, **297**, 528.

Rosendal, M., Fink, P., Bro, F., and Olesen, F. (2005). Somatization, heartsink patients, or functional somatic symptoms? Towards a clinical useful classification in primary health care. *Scandinavian Journal of Primary Health Care*, **23**, 3–10.

Salmon, P., Peters, S., and Stanley, I. (1999). Patients' perceptions of medical explanations for somatisation disorders: Qualitative analysis. *British Medical Journal*, **318**(7180), 372–376.

Salmon, P., Ring, A., Dowrick, C., and Humphris, G. (2005). What do general practice patients want when they present medically unexplained symptoms, and why do their doctors feel pressurized? *Journal of Psychosomatic Research*, **59**, 255–262.

Shapiro, R. (2008). *Suckers: How Alternative Medicine Makes Fools of Us All*. London: Harvill Secker.

Shohet, R. (2005). *Passionate Medicine: Making the Transition From Conventional Medicine to Homeopathy*. London and Philadelphia: Jessica Kingsley Publishers.

Shorter, E. (1992). *From Paralysis to Fatigue: A History of Psychosomatic Illness in the Modern Era*. New York: The Free Press.

Showalter, E. (1997). *Hystories: Hysterical Epidemics and Modern Media*. New York: Columbia University Press.

Singh, S. and Ernst, E. (2008). *Trick or Treatment: Alternative Medicine on Trial*. London: Bantam Press.

Stockl, A. (2007). Complex syndromes, ambivalent diagnosis, and existential uncertainty: The case of Systemic Lupus Erythematosus (SLE). *Social Science and Medicine*, **65**, 1549–1559.

Tovey, P. and Broom, A. (2007). Oncologists' and specialist cancer nurses' approaches to complemetary and alternative medicine and their impact on patient action. *Social Science and Medicine*, **64**, 2550–2564.

Zollman, C. and Vickers, C. (1999a). ABC of complementary medicine: Complementary medicine and the patient. *British Medical Journal*, **319**(7223), 1486–1489.

Zollman, C. and Vickers, C. (1999b). ABC of complementary medicine: Complementary medicine and the doctor. *British Medical Journal*, **319**(7224), 1558–1561.

CHAPTER 13

Talking about mistakes and dealing with complaints

Peter Washer

Learning points

This chapter will:

+ indicate the prevalence of medical errors and accidents (adverse events)

+ explain initiatives to promote patient safety

+ describe reasons why patients and relatives get angry and ways to calm volatile situations

+ describe what to do if a patient or relative complains.

The prevalence of medical errors and accidents (adverse events)

Everyone makes mistakes in their working life, and even with the best medical care in the world, there will still be occasions when things go wrong. Some medical errors will only lead to 'near misses', while others will result in medical accidents – injuries caused either as a result of misdiagnosis or by the medical treatment itself. When medical errors cause harm to patients, they are known as 'adverse events'. The phrase originates in pharmacology, where any unexpected or dangerous reaction to a drug is known as an adverse event. More generally in medicine, an adverse event has been defined as an *'injury resulting from a medical intervention (or omission), not the underlying condition of the patient'* (Kohn *et al.*, 2000). One study reviewed 1014 medical and nursing records from two acute London hospitals and found that 110 (10.8%) patients experienced an adverse event, with an overall rate of adverse events of 11.7% when multiple adverse events were included. A third of these led to at least a moderate disability or to death, and about a half of all these events were judged preventable with ordinary standards of care. Other studies in the USA and Australia suggest that from 3.7% to 16.6% of all patients experience an adverse event (Vincent et al., 2001).

However, accurately describing the prevalence of 'adverse' events is problematic for two reasons:

♦ The parameters of what counts as serious enough to be included in the definition varies (Vincent et al., 2001).

♦ The types of incident people usually think of as adverse events, for example medication administration errors, or a surgeon operating on the wrong side, are more common in acute care settings.

In the context of chronic illnesses, the focus is on trying to prevent or postpone 'adverse developments' that might unfold over an extended illness career (Lutfey & Freese, 2007).

Having acknowledged that it is difficult to be precise about how many adverse events occur, it is nevertheless clear that there is under-reporting of safety incidents (Vincent et al., 1999). In 2004, an online survey of 2575 UK doctors found that, although 80% of respondents had witnessed a colleague making a mistake, few were apparently willing to use the available systems to report it, and only 15% of serious incidents resulting in death or serious disability were reported (White, 2004).

Attitudes to adverse events

Several studies in the UK and USA have explored medical students' and doctors' attitudes to adverse events, and have looked at why doctors are reluctant to report them. Common factors that prevented reporting of adverse events were:

♦ a feeling that some adverse events are inevitable and unavoidable (Fischer et al., 2006; Waring, 2005)

♦ uncertainty as to which incidents need to be reported (Vincent et al., 1999)

♦ ambiguity and conflict about roles (for example between doctors and midwives) (Vincent et al., 1999)

♦ a concern that (junior) individuals would be blamed and reputations damaged (Vincent et al., 1999; Waring, 2005)

♦ not wanting to report mistakes made by more senior doctors (Fischer et al., 2006)

♦ a feeling that if a patient has not been harmed it is better not to draw attention to the error (Phitayakorn et al., 2008)

♦ a lack of trust in management (White, 2004)

♦ a lack of willingness to be regulated by non-doctors (Waring, 2005)

♦ a dislike of bureaucracy, which was associated with nursing rather than medicine (Waring, 2005)

♦ concerns that reporting would cause more work (Vincent et al., 1999; Waring, 2005).

Promoting patient safety

The problem with not reporting adverse events when they happen is that lessons cannot be learned from them, and this leaves patients vulnerable to the same mistakes happening again. Many observers attribute under-reporting to the punitive 'name and blame' approach that many healthcare organizations have taken to safety incidents. This culture discourages reporting and prevents organizational learning and improvement. We might contrast this culture of fear and subsequent under-reporting in medicine with the airline industry's non-punitive approach to reporting, which has been a significant contributory factor to its impressive safety record (Weiner, Hobgood & Lewis, 2008). For example, international research comparing attitudes to error, stress, and teamwork among healthcare staff in operating theatres and ICUs, and cockpit crew members found that the aviation industry's approach to errors was to deal with them non-punitively and pro-actively, while in medicine there were still substantial pressures to cover up mistakes (Sexton et al., 2000).

Some memory lapses and deviations from safe practice or standards may be the fault of one individual and are often associated with motivational problems such as low morale. However, most adverse events arise from organizational and systems failure (Taylor-Adams et al., 1999) such as:

♦ staff allocation problems

♦ poor supervision and management

♦ inadequate training

♦ high workload

♦ poor communication

♦ the use of medical locums and bank nurses

♦ inter-professional conflict

♦ equipment failures.

Policy changes to promote a no-blame or 'fair-blame' culture

In 2000, the US Institute of Medicine's Quality of Health-care in America Committee published a highly influential report called *To Err is Human* (Kohn *et al.*, 2000). One of its conclusions was that mistakes can be prevented by designing systems that make mistakes harder to make, for example by not stocking certain full-strength drugs that are toxic unless diluted. The report argued that individuals must still be careful and vigilant, and take responsibility for their actions. However, when an error did occur, blaming an individual did not make the system safer and prevent someone else from making the same mistake. The report argued for a change in the current culture of blame, which led to under-reporting of adverse events, to create a culture of safety (Jensen, 2008).

Safety experts argue that, to make incident reporting work, healthcare organizations must establish a 'just culture', in which health professionals feel assured that they will receive fair treatment when they report safety incidents – one in which individuals can report errors or near misses without fear of reprimand or reprisal, yet where those responsible for unsafe acts due to incompetence or recklessness will be held accountable (Weiner *et al.*, 2008).

To Err is Human had a profound impact in the USA and around the world, particularly in Australia (Depart-ment of Health NSW, 2007), and in the UK. In 2000, the UK Department of Health produced the report *An Organisation with a Memory* (Department of Health Expert Group, 2000), which was followed in 2002 by *Building a Safer NHS for Patients* (Department of Health, 2002), which set out the UK government's plans for promoting patient safety. A new mandatory reporting scheme for adverse events and 'near misses', was intro-duced, together with a new independent body, the UK National Patient Safety Agency (NPSA), to improve patient safety by collecting and analysing information on adverse events and producing solutions to prevent harm where risks were identified. The NPSA advice is that when a patient has been involved in a safety incident that led to them suffering harm, or to a relatives' death, the patient or their relatives should receive an apology and an explanation of what hap-pened (National Patient Safety Agency, 2005).

Why patients and relatives get angry

When patients and their relatives are dissatisfied with the care and treatment they receive, they can become angry, anxious, and distressed. Sometimes they may get angry even when things have not gone wrong with their medical or nursing care. This anger is a reaction to the helplessness they feel about their own or their loved one's illness. Anger can be a part of the grieving process, and can also be a reaction to loss or antici-pated loss. Anger can also be a manifestation of guilt, for example the not uncommon situation in which estranged relatives arrive at the bedside demanding that everything be done for the patient (von Gunten *et al.*, 2000). Guilt and grief are strong emotions that are sometimes expressed as anger, and this may be projected onto healthcare professionals, even when the individual professional is not at fault.

Ways to calm volatile situations

When people are angry, they often talk loudly and more quickly, and invade your personal space in a threaten-ing way. Use your communication skills to counter this – one natural reaction is to match their speed or volume of speech . . .

*butwhenyoutalkreallyfastyourvoiceinevitablygetssqueakyand
yousoundasifyou'restressedandoutofcontrolofthesituation* . . .

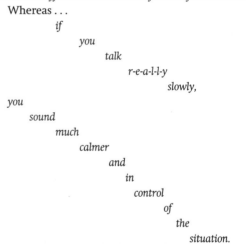

Another thing that happens if you slow your speech down is that your voice tends to get deeper, which gives you an air of *gravitas* that is quite difficult to pro-ject if you are talking quickly and sound squeaky. Try to keep calm, take a deep breath, and consciously talk slowly and softly.

Be aware of the effect that being on the receiving end of another person's anger can have on you. Even in simulated 'angry patient' consultations (with actors), students often get genuinely upset. Fight or flight responses are natural reactions, hot-wired into us through millions of years of evolution. When you are shouted at, it is normal to feel on the point of tears, to cry, to start shaking uncontrollably, or to feel suddenly angry yourself and want to lash out either verbally or physically. One UK study of 171 accident and emergency doctors found that one of the main causes of psychological distress for them was dealing with demanding, manipulative, violent, or aggressive patients (Williams *et al.*, 1997). If you feel overwhelmed by these types of feelings, remove yourself from the situation, take some time out, go somewhere quiet, and calm yourself down. Talk the situation through with your colleagues and seek support. Document the conversation in the patient's notes after you have discussed it with your colleagues and if the situation is serious enough, complete an incident form.

TIPS ON WHAT TO DO IF A PATIENT OR RELATIVE BECOMES ANGRY

♦ Think about your safety first – be aware of where the patient or relative is in relation to the door, just in case they become physically violent and you need to make a quick exit. Do not get physically 'fenced in'.

♦ Keep your distance. Not only is this a safety measure, but getting too close can make people feel uncomfortable and threatened.

♦ If possible, move the patient or relatives from public areas and go somewhere quiet – again be aware of safety and tell another member of staff where you are going.

♦ If possible, get the person to sit down. It is more difficult to keep up a pitch of anger when you are sitting than when you are standing.

♦ Allow them to vent their anger and do not interrupt. It is very difficult to keep on shouting for an extended period.

♦ Consciously use the tone, speed, and volume of your speech to calm the person.

♦ Acknowledge their distress: '**I can see how upset you are.**'

♦ Apologize (see below): '**I'm really sorry this has happened to you.**'

♦ Empathize, both verbally – '**I would feel the same in your situation**' – and non-verbally with your body language (nodding, eye contact, looking concerned).

♦ Say what you will do to try and clarify what has happened, and if possible to put it right.

♦ Try not to get defensive or sarcastic.

♦ Try to avoid mirroring the person's pitch, pace, tone of voice, or body language.

♦ Telling an emotional or angry person, '**Calm down**' or, '**Don't worry**' is likely to have the opposite effect.

♦ Try to avoid colluding with the patient or relatives or criticizing your colleagues. Say something like: '**I can't really comment on the medical details because I need to find out about what happened from the other doctors, but I'll try to find out for you.**'

♦ Try to avoid matching the person's anger or showing them if you are upset. If you can feel this starting to happen, remove yourself from the situation. Say: '**I'm sorry, but I need to stop this conversation now. I'll talk to you again later**', and leave.

When patients and relatives are angry, they will often threaten to complain. If this happens, try to avoid getting defensive. Try to open the conversation out rather than close it down. Acknowledge calmly that they can complain if they want to and that you will tell them how to go about it if they decide that is want they want to do. Then say that first it is important to be clear about what happened, what the issues are, and what can be done to put them right. Emphasize what is being done for the patient, offer to facilitate a second opinion, reinforce the message that everyone wants the best care for them, and try to suggest ways that everyone can work together to make that happen (von Gunten *et al.*, 2000).

Complaints and litigation

Complaints, apologies, and explanations

Patients' and relatives' disappointment and anger about the care they have or have not received can often be mollified though effective communication skills – giving them a full explanation of events, an apology, and an assurance that steps have been taken to ensure the same thing will not happen to anyone else. When these measures do not work, a formal complaint may follow. Complaints often follow adverse events, but not all complaints are the result of an adverse event, and, similarly, not all adverse events lead to a complaint (Cave & Dacre, 2008).

In the UK, patients or relatives can complain both through the National Health Service complaints procedure and, if they have complaints about a specific doctor, they can complain to the General Medical Council. Complaints about medical students are unusual, but if a complaint were to arise from your involvement in a patient's care while you were still a student, the complaint would be handled in line with the usual complaints procedure. You are unlikely to be asked to respond to the complainant directly, but you might be asked to provide information to your supervisor or consultant to enable the hospital Trust to respond (Kirkpatrick, 2004).

When a patient complains, or even asks to see their notes, often the hospital or service provider responds by closing down avenues of communication, fearing that anything they say may make them vulnerable because of the threat of litigation. This usually leads to patients and relatives becoming even more frustrated and angry. They begin to form a (correct) impression that there is a conspiracy of silence against them or that there must therefore be something to hide. This can lead to the conflict escalating and spinning out of the control of both sides. One of the factors that inhibits doctors and other staff from apologizing is the fear that this will be taken as an admission of liability in future possible court action. The NHS Litigation Authority is quite clear on this point:

'It seems to us that it is both natural and desirable for those involved in treatment which produces an adverse result, for whatever reason, to sympathize with the patient or the patient's relatives and to express sorrow or regret at the outcome. Such expressions of regret would not normally constitute an admission of liability, either in part or full, and it is not our policy to prohibit them, nor to dispute any payment, under any scheme, solely on the grounds of such an expression of regret' (NHS Litigation Authority, 2007).

If a patient wants an explanation of what has happened, or asks to see their notes, then remember that nothing is likely to be revealed that would not subsequently be disclosed in the event of litigation (NHS Litigation Authority, 2007). This underlines the point made about written information earlier in this book. When writing about patients, whether in their paper or electronic records or in a letter to another healthcare professional, never write anything that you would not be happy for the patient or their relatives to read.

PODCAST

A patient's perspective

"So when you went to see the solicitor that was the goal, to get your notes?"

"Yeah, just to find out what had happened."

"Right, and what happened when you . . . how long did it take to . . ."

". . . it took my solicitor 6 months to get my notes. Then we had to have them translated so that I could understand them, and then it was obvious that things had gone wrong. My solicitor advised me to sue them. I didn't want to sue them, I just wanted an explanation. I couldn't get an explanation from them, so I ended up suing them."

. . .

"If there'd been a proper explanation before you got to the solicitor, then the whole thing wouldn't have spun in that direction [of litigation]?"

"No, of course not. When I first rung up the hospital and asked what had happened to me, if they'd just explained what had happened to me, that would've been that. You know, a year of lying in bed, trying to recover, and not knowing what had actually been done to me. I've got all these scars and wounds and I didn't know what they were for."

Podcast – Peter Kemble, who sued his hospital, and eventually received an out-of-court settlement

Litigation and redress

Ultimately, if the patient and relatives are not satisfied with any explanation and apology given arising from their complaint, then they can resort to litigation, although, in the UK context at least, very few do. Most of the clinical negligence cases that are started are either abandoned by the complainants or are settled before they go to court. Clinical negligence cases usually take many years to reach a resolution, and they are financially very costly for both complainant and the hospital involved. More importantly, however, they are also costly in terms of the stress caused to all parties.

Research indicates that at the root of most litigation against doctors is poor clinical communication skills, both between doctors and patients and inter-professionally, rather than poor clinical practice. For example, one UK study of 227 patients and relatives who were taking legal action (this study was mentioned in Chapter 1) found that complainants often blamed doctors not so much for the original mistakes, but for a lack of openness or willingness to explain. They complained that the poor care extended well beyond the original incident. They suffered an absence of explanations, a lack of honesty, and a reluctance to apologize, or were treated as neurotic. Where explanations were given, they were seldom thought to be clear or sufficiently informative. In most cases, these secondary problems contributed to their decision to take legal action (Vincent *et al.*, 1994).

Another US study examined 60 surgical malpractice claims cases involving communication breakdowns and found that the most common problems involved junior doctors failing to notify the attending surgeon of critical events and a failure to attend to handovers. Situations where one professional had substantially more power and greater rank than another, and ambiguity about responsibilities, were common associated factors. Commonly, information was never passed on, or was communicated but inaccurately received (Greenberg *et al.*, 2007).

Summary

Doctors have a high degree of professional autonomy and tend to be competitive high achievers. The individualist culture of medicine has tended to place less importance on team working and organizational efficiency. As a result, it is often difficult for doctors to admit their own mistakes. In the culture of the medical profession, it is often regarded as unprofessional to criticize the poor practice of other doctors. Therefore, mistakes, errors, and adverse events frequently go unreported, leaving the opportunity for the same mistakes to happen again, perhaps with more serious consequences next time. Many countries have now introduced initiatives to encourage adverse event reporting, and thus promote patient safety. Sometimes adverse events or other circumstances can lead to patients and relatives getting angry and complaining about their care. Effective communication skills can often defuse these situations, and being open and offering a detailed explanation and apology may in many instances be the end of the matter. A small minority of patients who are not satisfied with the results of a complaint will initiate litigation.

Further reading

The UK National Patient Safety Agency has produced a reference guide dealing with how to respond when a patient has been harmed.

National Patient Safety Agency (2005). *Being Open When Patients Are Harmed*. London: NPSA.

This guide is available online – the link can be found at the Online Resource Centre for this book.

Visit the Online Resource Centre for *Clinical Communication Skills* at: www.oxfordtextbooks.co.uk/orc/washer

References

Cave, J. and Dacre, J. (2008). Dealing with complaints. *British Medical Journal*, **336**, 326–336.

Department of Health (2002). *Building a Safer NHS for Patients: Implementing an Organisation with a Memory*. London: HMSO.

Department of Health Expert Group (2000). *An Organisation with a Memory*. London: HMSO.

Department of Health NSW (2007). *Open Disclosure Guidelines*. North Sydney, NSW: Department of Health, NSW.

Fischer, M., Mazor, K., Baril, J., Alper, E., DeMarco, D., and Pugnaire, M. (2006). Learning from mistakes. *Journal of General Internal Medicine*, **21**, 419–423.

Greenberg, C., Regenbogen, S., Studdert, D., Lipsitz, S., Rogers, S., Zinner, M., and Gawande, A. (2007). Patterns of communication breakdowns resulting in injury to surgical patients. *Journal of the American College of Surgeons*, **204**(4), 533–540.

Jensen, C. (2008). Sociology, systems and (patient) safety: Knowledge translations in health policy. *Sociology of Health and Illness*, **30**(2), 309–324.

Kirkpatrick, A. (2004). Resolving complaints. *Student British Medical Journal*, **12**, 89–132.

Kohn, L., Corrigan, J., and Donaldson, M. (2000). *To Err is Human – Building a Safer Health System*. Washington, DC: Institute of Medicine, National Academy Press.

Lutfey, K. and Freese, J. (2007). Ambiguities of chronic illness management and challenges to the medical error paradigm. *Social Science and Medicine*, **64**, 314–325.

National Patient Safety Agency (2005). *Being Open When Patients Are Harmed*. London: National Patient Safety Agency.

NHS Litigation Authority (2007). *Apologies and Explanations*. London: NHS Litigation Authority.

Phitayakorn, R., Williams, R., Yudkowsky, R., Harris, I., Hauge, L., Widmann, W., Sullivan, M., and Mellinger,

J. (2008). Patient-care-related telephone communication between general surgery residents and attending surgeons. *Journal of the American College of Surgeons*, **206**(4), 742–750.

Sexton, J., Thomas, E., and Helmreich, R. (2000). Error, stress, and teamwork in medicine and aviation: Cross sectional surveys. *British Medical Journal*, **320**(7237), 745–749.

Taylor-Adams, S., Vincent, C., and Stanhope, N. (1999). Applying human factors methods to the investigation and analysis of clinical adverse events. *Safety Science*, **31**, 143–159.

Vincent, C., Young, A., and Phillips, A. (1994). Why do patients sue doctors? A study of patients and relatives taking legal action. *The Lancet*, **343**(8913), 1609–1613.

Vincent, C., Stanhope, N., and Crowley-Murphey, M. (1999). Reasons for not reporting adverse events: An empirical study. *Journal of Evaluation in Clinical Practice*, **5**(1), 13–21.

Vincent, C., Neale, G., and Woloshynowych, M. (2001). Adverse events in British hospitals: Preliminary retrospective record review. *British Medical Journal*, **322**(7285), 517–519.

von Gunten, C., Ferris, F., and Emanuel, L. (2000). Ensuring competency in end-of-life care: Communication and relational skills. *Journal of the American Medical Association*, **284**(23), 3051–3057.

Waring, J. (2005). Beyond blame: Cultural barriers to medical incident reporting. *Social Science and Medicine*, **60**, 1927–1935.

Weiner, B., Hobgood, C., and Lewis, M. (2008). The meaning of justice in safety incident reporting. *Social Science and Medicine*, **66**, 403–413.

White, C. (2004). Doctors mistrust systems for reporting medical mistakes. *British Medical Journal*, **329**(7456), 12–13.

Williams, S., Dale, J., Glucksman, E., and Wellesley, A. (1997). Senior house officers' work related stressors, psychological distress, and confidence in performing clinical tasks in accident and emergency: A questionnaire study. *British Medical Journal*, **314**(7082), 713–718.

CHAPTER 14

Shared decision making and communicating risk

Peter Washer

Learning points

This chapter will:

♦ clarify the notion of shared decision making

♦ discuss the ethics of communicating risk

♦ describe some tools to help shared decision making by translating statistical data into information that patients can use to inform their decisions.

If we reflect on the complexity of modern medicine, it is perhaps not surprising that patients often feel over-whelmed by the information that they need to process in order to decide what is best for them. Think of the range of investigations and treatments available today, and the research evidence available to support them, and compare that with what would have been available to patients even a couple of generations ago, say at the end of the Second World War. Another change in the context of contemporary medical practice is that society is ever more risk-aware and people are more risk-averse. The furore over the alleged link between autism and the measles, mumps, and rubella (MMR) vaccination in the 1990s is one example (Bellaby, 2003). Patients also have access to a great deal more information now through the Internet, and many patients can rightly be called experts, particularly some patients with chronic medical conditions or diseases like AIDS.

Into this culture of increasing medical sophistication, heightened risk-awareness and greater access to information, a further element in the social context of medical practice is a greater focus on patient autonomy. There is a move away from the paternalistic 'doctor knows best' model of the doctor–patient relationship, towards informed consent, partnership, and shared decision-making models. Medicolegally, in order for a patient to give a valid consent for an investigation or treatment, they need to be able to understand and weigh up the potential risks and benefits of the different courses of action. However, patients cannot exercise their autonomy unless they understand the statistics as they are presented. Therefore, doctors need to be able to explain and interpret complex information for patients in such a way so that they can understand the options available to them, and then, together with their doctors, arrive at a decision.

This chapter will consider these issues and provide some guidance on how best to present complex statistical information so that patients can actively participate in the medical decision-making process.

Shared decision making

The key elements of the shared decision-making model are that:

1 At least two parties are involved, doctor and patient, although in reality patients' relatives and friends may have a part to play, and more than one doctor may participate, for example a surgeon and an oncologist in the case of cancer.

2 Both parties share information.

3 Both parties try to build a consensus about the preferred treatment.

4 An agreement is reached on the treatment to be implemented (Charles, Gafni & Whelan, 1997).

A review of the research into shared decision making concluded that, although its benefits were not yet clearly demonstrated, generally patients want to be informed of treatment alternatives and to be involved in treatment decisions (Guadagnoli & Ward, 1998). For example, one Australian study of 233 cancer patients and their oncologists suggests that encouraging participation in decision making may be the best standard approach. Patients who reported shared roles in decision making were most satisfied with the consultation, and those who reported that either themselves or the doctor exclusively made the decision were least satisfied (Gattellari et al., 2001).

However, although on the face of it this model seems sound, in practice there may be barriers to implementing it. For example, one UK study of 62 GP consultations found little evidence that doctors and patients participate in the way described by Charles et al. (1997). The first two of the four conditions said to be necessary for shared decision making were not generally present, so there was no basis on which to build a consensus about the preferred method of treatment, and to reach an agreement on which treatment to implement. Even when information was shared, patients' beliefs were not taken seriously. The GPs identified a number of barriers to sharing decision making, including time pressures, and the doctors' perception that patients would not understand medical language and concepts (Stevenson et al., 2000). Another UK study interviewed 39 GPs and found that they felt they did not have sufficient information to explain the risks and benefits of treatment choices. They were concerned about sharing the uncertainties about the outcomes of medical treatments, and causing anxiety by exposing patients to the fact that data are often unavailable or unknown. The doctors admitted using 'friendly persuasion' as their usual practice (Elwyn et al., 1999a).

Screening programmes

Many diseases, such as different types of cancer, have screening programmes, which aim to find people who are at higher risk of a disease and test them before symptoms appear, in order to detect early stages of the disease and offer effective early treatment. The problems associated with shared decision making and communicating risk are important enough when they relate to medical treatments, when a choice has to be made about the best treatment to treat or cure the patient's disease. However, the issues come into even sharper focus when dealing with screening programmes for people who are not ill.

Screening programmes for different diseases have to meet certain criteria:

◆ They must be directed towards a specific disease and a target population.

◆ The progression of the disease must be well understood.

◆ Importantly, an effective treatment or intervention must already be available.

Some genetic tests are truly diagnostic – for example if a person has the specific disease-causing sequence of DNA that causes Huntingdon's disease, then a genetic test will tell with 100% certainty that they will get the disease; there are no false positives or false negatives.

This level of certainty is extremely rare, however, and most tests can only tell whether a person is *likely* to get a disease in the future. Predictive or susceptibility tests are about likelihood, not certainty (Sense About Science, 2008). Patient materials and the media frequently report statistics about screening tests for maximum impact, in particular by reporting relative risks instead of absolute ones (see below), which research indicates has the greatest effect on influencing uptake of screening (Edwards *et al.*, 2001).

You might think 'What could be the harm in that?' Screening programmes such as mammography may cause inconvenience and temporary anxiety while waiting for the results of further tests when there is a false-positive result, but set against that, what of the lives saved? However, mammography screening can lead to unnecessary biopsies arising from over-diagnosis, where 'biopsy' may mean segmental excisions, mastectomy, radiotherapy, and subsequent endocrine treatments (Thornton *et al.*, 2003). In addition, one in five 'cancers' detected by mammograms in the NHS Breast Screening Programme are ductal carcinoma *in situ*, a non-invasive condition in which abnormal cells are found in the lining of a breast duct but have not spread to other tissues in the breast. In some cases, ductal carcinoma *in situ* may become invasive and spread, but it is not possible to predict accurately which of these cancers will become invasive. Approximately half of those detected will never progress to an invasive cancer, and some others will even regress.

These complexities and subtleties regarding testing and screening are often not presented to patients. Statistical and risk information needs to be given in a format that is as clear as possible, so that patients and their doctors can make the decision that is the right one for that particular patient. The last section of this chapter describes various ways of doing this.

Ethics and risk communication

There is little certainty in medicine, and no such thing as medicine that is risk free. Every treatment and investigation carries some degree of risk, as well as the potential for benefit. Even if there were medical certainties, there would still be no such thing as a *purely medical* decision, or only one best treatment. There will always be at least one other treatment option – namely non-treatment. A decision made on *purely medical* grounds cannot take into account a patient's preferences and values, which may not correspond with

their doctor's. To make consent fully patient-centred, doctors need to first ask what patients want from treatment. Patients who want to share decisions find it easier to do so if the process begins with an exploration of their objectives (Bridson *et al.*, 2003).

PODCAST

A patient's perspective

"Initially I saw the consultant as a result of conversations with the breast care nurse in relation to assisted fertility issues, because as I said I was just about to get married, I hadn't any children and we had been planning on starting a family, though I saw the consultant to put the issues of my treatment in the context of fertility, assisted fertility issues . . . The options offered to me were . . . I had them presented to me in terms of the success rate, as a result of surgery, surgery plus radiotherapy, surgery plus radiotherapy and hormone treatment, because the cancer was an oestrogen-based tumour, or surgery, radiotherapy and chemotherapy."

". . . so increasing in the success rates, the latter ones being the highest?"

"Yes, I mean the success rate, if I had selected the option of chemotherapy combined with radiotherapy and surgery was 1% greater than if I had gone for the hormone-based treatment combined with radiotherapy and surgery, but then it was put in the context of far fewer extreme side effects."

"Sure, so did you come away from that consultation with the sense that the doctor and the breast care team were favouring a particular option?"

"Yes, I did. I felt they were favouring the hormone-based treatment combined with radiotherapy and surgery because it had a higher success rate. I think at the time they said it had 95%, but it had far fewer side effects than if I had opted for the chemotherapy, which had a slightly, I think a 1%, higher success rate but significantly more side effects, so I came away feeling that was the option that was being sort of highly recommended, *but it was still put in the context of it being my choice.*"

Podcast – Roisin, 41-year-old woman with breast cancer

Often people talk about the relative 'effectiveness' of different ways of presenting risk information. In this context, 'effective' usually means getting patients to agree with what the doctor believes is in the patient's best interests. Many might argue that there is nothing wrong with this if it produces the 'right' outcome. Is it not a good thing that children are vaccinated against MMR? Is it not better if people stop smoking? Health educators used to hold the view that they should use these 'effective' presentations of information to promote the treatment options and screening programmes that were beneficial according to established medical opinion (Edwards & Elwyn, 2001). Research on patient information materials indicates that information is often presented in such a way as to promote a particular outcome. However, that information is often inaccurate, gives an over-optimistic view, and fails to mention that there is more than one option, the effects of no treatment, or any scientific uncertainties, and variation in clinical opinion. While benefits of tests and treatments are emphasized, often any risks of harm, limitations, and side effects are glossed over (Coulter *et al.*, 1999; Godolphin *et al.*, 2001; Thornton *et al.*, 2003). Interestingly, research indicates that improved patient knowledge as a result of receiving more information that is understandable to the patient is associated with a subsequent greater wariness to take treatments or participate in trials (Edwards *et al.*, 2001).

Tools for facilitating shared decision making

Sharing information is not the same thing as sharing decision making. In order to participate in the decision-making process, patients first need to understand the information that is presented to them. The following sections provide a range of evidence-based means of facilitating this.

Use decision aids

One way to help patients to clarify their values concerning benefits and harms is to use patient decision aids, which explain options, quantify risks and benefits, and provide structured guidance. These are available in paper format, on DVD, and online (see the Online Resource Centre for this book for web links). They have been implemented successfully in specialist clinics in the UK and Canada, and in primary care clinics in the USA (Stacey *et al.*, 2008). Research shows that the use of decision aids produces better knowledge of options and outcomes, although they do not necessarily reduce anxiety (O'Connor *et al.*, 1999).

Use absolute risks instead of relative risks

If you said, **'Mammography screening reduces a woman's risk of dying from breast cancer by 25%'**, most people would interpret the 25% reduction as referring to women who undergo mammography screening, and think that if they undergo mammography their chances of dying of breast cancer were reduced by a quarter. In fact, the relative risk being described here relates to a different category of women, namely those who die of breast cancer without being screened (Gigerenzer & Edwards, 2003). Representing this information in the form of a table makes this point clear:

Mammography reduces breast cancer mortality by 25%	
Treatment	**Deaths per 1000 women**
No mammography screening	4
Mammography screening	3

If you do not screen women by mammography, there will be four deaths. If you do screen, three will die. Therefore, for every 1000 treated there will be one less death. If we describe this risk in terms of absolute risks, it becomes easier to understand: '*In every 1000 women who undergo screening, one will be saved from dying of breast cancer.*' Or we can use the number needed to treat: '*To prevent one death from breast cancer, 1000 women need to undergo screening for 10 years*' (Gigerenzer & Edwards, 2003).

Another useful way to present this information would be to use frequency diagrams (see below).

Use natural frequencies

The chance of a particular screening test, such as a mammogram or prostate-specific antigen test, producing a positive test result and detecting people with the disease is known as the sensitivity of the test. The specificity of a test is the chance of a test excluding people who do not have the disease, by giving a negative test result. Sensitivity and specificity are usually communicated as conditional probabilities, but like the relative risk reduction, conditional probabilities are confusing because they make it difficult to understand what class of events a percentage refers to.

Most people would assume that a positive result from a mammogram would mean that a woman did indeed have breast cancer. Yet this does not take account of the sensitivity of the test. Gigerenzer & Edwards (2003) give the following example:

'*The probability that a woman has breast cancer is 0.8%. If she does have breast cancer, the probability that a mammogram will show a positive result is 90%. If a woman does not have breast cancer, the probability of a positive result is 7%.*

If a woman has a positive mammogram, what then is the probability she actually has breast cancer?'

If we present this example in terms of natural frequencies rather than in terms of conditional probabilities, it becomes much easier to understand:

'The probability that a woman has breast cancer is 0.8%.'

In other words, eight out of every 1000 women have breast cancer. [This is the prevalence of the disease, which is the number of people (alive) with a condition in a given population on a certain date, and is usually expressed as a percentage. The incidence of a disease is the number of people newly diagnosed with a condition in a specific time period, and is expressed as a number.]

'If she does have breast cancer, the probability that a mammogram will show a positive result is 90%.'

In other words, of these eight women, seven will have a positive result on mammography, which is the sensitivity of the test.

'If a woman does not have breast cancer, the probability of a positive result is 7%.'

So, of the 992 (1000 − 8) women who do not have breast cancer, 7% (of 992), or roughly 69 women, will still have positive mammograms, which is the false-positive rate.

Therefore, of the 69 women who have a positive mammogram, only seven will actually have breast cancer. Expressed as a percentage, this is 7/(7 + 69) or roughly 9%. In fact then, the chances of a woman who tests positive on mammography actually having breast cancer are about one in ten.

Use frequency statements

Single-event probabilities such as, **'You have a 25% chance of getting this side effect from this medicine'** can be confusing. Some people might think this meant that a quarter of people taking the medicine get the side effect, while other people might think it meant that you would get that side effect a quarter of the times you took it. Using frequency statements can help people to visualize the risk. For example: **'Imagine 100 people like you taking this medicine; 25 of them can expect to get this side effect, but the other 75 won't.'**

Use consistent denominators

If you said to many people, **'If we treat your condition you have an 89 in 100 chance of improvement, but the treatment carries a 1 in 25 risk of complications'**, they might not be clear which option carries the lower risk,

because of the different denominators used. If you use the same denominator in both cases, it becomes clearer. For example: **'89 out of 100 people with your condition who have treatment will get better, but four in 100 people can expect to have complications.'**

Avoid using terms such as 'high' or 'low' risk

The terms 'high risk' or 'low risk' are vague and open to a wide interpretation. In addition, categorizing people as being at 'high risk' of something may lead them to become overly worried and demotivated to change their behaviour, whereas people told they are at 'low risk' of something could be falsely reassured (Edwards *et al.*, 1998). It has been suggested that there should be a standardized language of risk, in which certain terms equate to particular frequencies, such as 'high' for over 1 in 100, or 'moderate' for 1 in 1000 and so on (Calman & Royston, 1997), although there seems little enthusiasm for this approach among doctors. Therefore, it is probably best to avoid classifying risks as 'high' or 'low'.

Frame the risk both positively and negatively

If you frame a risk positively, for example, **'You have an 80% chance of not having any complications from this operation'**, then a patient is more likely to agree to it than if the risk is framed negatively, as in, **'You have a 20% chance of developing postoperative complications.'** We should not be trying to manipulate the patient's decision either way, so the ethical solution is to present the risk both positively and negatively, for example, **'Out of every 100 people who have this operation, 20 develop a postoperative complication, but 80 do not have any problems.'**

Present information visually

Research indicates that graphical displays of information are useful for some patients, particularly simple bar charts (Edwards *et al.*, 2002), but it is important that the same scales are used on any graphs or charts to avoid confusion (Thomson *et al.*, 2005).

Another visual way to present statistics that may help people understand is by frequency diagrams. Gigerenzer and Edwards (2003) give the following example:

'The standard test for colorectal cancer is the faecal occult blood test (FOTB). For symptom-free people over 50 screened using this test, the probability that one of these people has colorectal cancer (the prevalence of the disease) is 0.3%. If they do have cancer, there is a 50% probability that they will have a positive FOTB (the sensitivity of the test). If they don't, the

probability of a (false) positive test is 3%. Imagine a person over 50 with no symptoms who has a positive FOTB test. What is the probability that they have cancer?'

On the basis of this information as presented, most people would find it difficult to work out the answer. However, if we present this same data as a diagram (**Figure 14.1**), it becomes much easier to see what is going on.

Thirty out of every 10,000 people have colorectal cancer. Of these 30 people, 15 will have a positive FOTB test result. Of the remaining 9970 people without cancer, 300 will still have a positive FOTB, no doubt leading to heightened anxiety when they do not in fact have the disease. Of the 315 people who have a positive test, only 15 have cancer, which is a probability of 4.8% or 1 in 20. So in other words, roughly five out of every 100 positive FOTB tests are false positives, so the chances of a person with a positive FOTB result actually having colorectal cancer are 1 in 20.

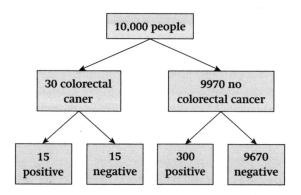

Figure 14.1 Frequency diagram for the Faecal occult blood test (FOTB)

Use time frames and compare medical with non-medical risks

One way to contextualize a risk is to give the chance of the risk of something happening over the course of a lifetime, or over a 5-year or 10-year time scale (Edwards *et al.*, 2002; Thomson *et al.*, 2005). Another way to contextualize the risk associated with a medical treatment is to compare it with other medical and non-medical risks. For example, you might compare the risk of a patient's chance of dying of a particular cancer with other people's risk of getting the same cancer, or with the patient's chance of dying of other cancers, or with other common causes of death in general, such

as road accidents. There are risk calculators available to help you do this via the Online Resource Centre for this book.

TOOLS TO HELP TRANSLATE STATISTICAL DATA INTO MORE EASILY UNDERSTOOD INFORMATION THAT PATIENTS CAN USE TO INFORM THEIR DECISIONS

♦ Use absolute risks or actual numbers

♦ Use natural frequencies

♦ Use frequency statements

♦ Use consistent denominators

♦ Frame the risk both positively and negatively

♦ Present information visually using charts and frequency diagrams

♦ Use time frames and lifetime risks, and compare medical with non-medical risks

♦ As far as possible, use individualized or tailored risk estimates

♦ Avoid deliberately presenting data in such a way as might manipulate a decision one way or another

♦ Contextualize any relative risks, conditional probabilities (such as sensitivity and specificity), or single-event probabilities

♦ Avoid descriptive terms such as 'high' or 'low' risk

Use individualized risk estimates

Individualized risk estimates are based on formulae derived from epidemiological data and estimate a person's own risk factors for a condition, using information such as their age and family history. Web-based risk calculators are available that can calculate quantitative risk estimates for various diseases such as breast cancer, lung cancer, and myocardial infarction (again, see the Online Resource Centre). However, most only calculate the chance of developing a particular disease, not of dying of it, nor do they give any sense of the uncertainty inherent in risk calculations (Woloshin *et al.*, 2003). Also, bear in mind that improvements in treatments and earlier diagnosis continue to improve survival rates for many diseases.

Summary

Faced with an increasingly complex range of medical interventions, patients should be encouraged to consider good evidence with their doctor in order to inform their shared decision making. Information needs to be presented in ways that are most easily understood. Doctors should not aim to influence patient decisions, but should explore the significance of the risk with their individual patients. Doctor and patient can then jointly reach the best decision for that particular patient, bearing in mind the particular patient's preferences and life circumstances, as well as the medical details of the disease and treatment options available.

Further reading

The most accessible book on effective ways to communicate statistics is:

Gigerenzer, G. (2002). *Reckoning with Risk: Learning to Live with Uncertainty*. London: Penguin.

Visit the Online Resource Centre for *Clinical Communication Skills* at: www.oxfordtextbooks.co.uk/orc/washer, which includes links to many relevant websites that provide a range of tools to help inform doctor and patient decision making.

References

Bellaby, P. (2003). Communication and miscommunication of risk: Understanding UK parents' attitudes to combined MMR vaccination. *British Medical Journal*, **327**(7417), 725–728.

Bridson, J., Hammond, C., Leach, A., and Chester, M. (2003). Making consent patient centred. *British Medical Journal*, **327**(7424), 1159–1161.

Calman, K. and Royston, G. (1997). Risk language and dialects. *British Medical Journal*, **315**(7113), 939–942.

Charles, C., Gafni, A., and Whelan, T. (1997). Shared decision-making in the medical encounter: What does it mean? (or it takes at least two to tango). *Social Science and Medicine*, **44**(5), 681–692.

Coulter, A., Entwistle, V., & Gilbert, D. (1999). Sharing decisions with patients: Is the information good enough? *British Medical Journal*, **318**(7179), 318–322.

Edwards, A. and Elwyn, G.J. (2001). Risks – Listen and don't mislead. *British Journal of General Practice*, **51**(465), 259–260.

Edwards, A., Matthews, E., Pill, R., and Bloor, M. (1998). Communication about risk: The responses of primary care professionals to standardizing the 'language of

risk' and communication tools. *Family Practice*, **15**(4), 301–307.

Edwards, A., Elwyn, G., Covey, J., Matthews, E., and Pill, R. (2001). Presenting risk information – A review of the effects of 'framing' and other manipulations on patient outcomes. *Journal of Health Communication*, **6**(1), 61–82.

Edwards, A., Elwyn, G., and Mulley, A. (2002). Explaining risks: Turning numerical data into meaningful pictures. *British Medical Journal*, **324**(7341), 827–830.

Elwyn, G., Edwards, A., Gwyn, R., and Grol, R. (1999a). Towards a feasible model for shared decision making: Focus group study with general practice registrars. *British Medical Journal*, **319**(7212), 753–756.

Gattellari, M., Butow, P.N., and Tattersall, M.H. (2001). Sharing decisions in cancer care. *Social Science and Medicine*, **52**(12), 1865–1878.

Gigerenzer, G. and Edwards, A. (2003). Simple tools for understanding risks: From innumeracy to insight. *British Medical Journal*, **327**(7417), 741–744.

Godolphin, W., Towle, A., and McKendry, R. (2001). Evaluation of the quality of patient information to support informed shared decision making. *Health Expectations*, **4**(4), 235–242.

Guadagnoli, E. and Ward, P. (1998). Patient participation in decision-making. *Social Science and Medicine*, **47**(3), 329–339.

O'Connor, A.M., Rostom, A., Fiset, V., Tetroe, J., Entwistle, V., Llewellyn-Thomas, H., Holmes-Rovner, M., Barry, M., and Jones, J. (1999). Decision aids for patients facing health treatment or screening decisions: Systematic review. *British Medical Journal*, **319**(7212), 731–734.

Sense About Science (2008). *Making Sense of Testing: A Guide to Why Scans and Health Tests For Well People Aren't Aways a Good Idea*. London: Sense About Science.

Stacey, D., Hawker, G., Dervin, G., Tomek, I., Cochran, N., Tugwell, P., and O'Connor, A.M. (2008). Improving shared decision making in osteoarthritis. *British Medical Journal*, **336**(650), 954–955.

Stevenson, F.A., Barry, C.A., Britten, N., Barber, N., and Bradley, C.P. (2000). Doctor–patient communication about drugs: The evidence for shared decision making. *Social Science and Medicine*, **50**(6), 829–840.

Thomson, R., Edwards, A., and Grey, J. (2005). Risk communication in the clinical consultation. *Clinical Medicine*, **5**(5), 465–469.

Thornton, H., Edwards, A., and Baum, M. (2003). Women need better information about routine mammography. *British Medical Journal*, **327**(7406), 101–103.

Woloshin, S., Schwartz, L., and Ellner, A. (2003). Making sense of risk information on the web: Don't forget the basics. *British Medical Journal*, **327**(7417), 695–696.

CHAPTER 15

Breaking bad news

Judith Cave

Learning points

This chapter will:

- explain how to tell patients bad news
- discuss coping strategies to deal with the aftermath when another professional has broken bad news
- help you deal with your own emotions.

When you are taught how to break bad news as a medical student, the focus is often on shocking news such as a new cancer diagnosis or sudden death. In reality, students and junior doctors often break news that is less extreme but is still highly upsetting for patients, for example news of cancelled operations, long waits for investigations, or delayed hospital discharges. Even a postponed operation may have far-ranging effects on a patient's social life, employment (especially if they are self-employed), holidays, trust in the healthcare team, and of course physical health. It is impossible to judge in advance the effect any piece of news will have on a patient, and often news will have wider negative implications than you might have been able to anticipate (Eggly *et al.*, 2006).

Breaking bad news is a team effort, so although a consultant may actually deliver the news, as a medical student you have your part to play in helping to support the patient (Wittenberg-Lyles *et al.*, 2008). As a junior doctor, you are likely to have to break bad news yourself. Evidence shows that within their first year of qualifying, 79% of doctors break bad news to a patient at least once, 92% are asked questions by patients that initiate discussion of bad news, and 96% break bad news to relatives of a patient (Schildmann *et al.*, 2005).

This chapter covers breaking bad news, dealing with the aftermath of that news, and taking a team-based approach to supporting both the patient and yourself. The advice should be relevant to any consultation involving imparting difficult information; the principles of breaking bad news are core skills for any healthcare professional.

How to tell patients bad news

In the past, doctors tended to try to protect patients by hiding bad news or by using euphemisms. Evidence shows, however, that 98% of patients want their doctors to be realistic (Hagerty *et al.*, 2005). Patients want information about their condition and their outlook, even when the news is bad; for example, in a large study of 2231 cancer patients, 87% wanted as much information as possible – good or bad – and 98% wanted to know if they had cancer (Jenkins *et al.*, 2001).

A bad news consultation involves preparation (if possible) and follow-up. Preparation means not only thinking about the news itself but about the patient, any support available, the physical surroundings, and your own state of mind and workload. During the consultation, you will need to consider what the patient knows and understands already, how to deliver the news, and how to support the patient through any reaction they have. You will also need to end the consultation by establishing a mutually agreed plan for dealing with the problem. This section talks you through the process of breaking bad news in detail. In practice, you will find that different bits of advice are relevant for different situations.

Preparing yourself

Many doctors dread breaking bad news, being fearful of how patients will react (Dosanjh *et al.*, 2001). This may lead them to procrastinate, worrying that the patient will blame them or that their relationship with the patient will be damaged. In fact, there is no evidence that patients 'shoot the messenger' (Barnett, 2002). However, it is not always wise to rush in immediately with a piece of news. Timing is important, as well as having the full picture. When you are a junior doctor, if you are in doubt about whether to tell a patient something, talk it through with a senior colleague first.

Before the consultation, run through in your mind exactly what information needs to be conveyed and what the implications of that news might be from the patient's perspective. Also think about what questions the patient is most likely to ask and whether you have the answers. If you do not have all the information you need, consider whether you should delay the consultation and seek advice.

One practical thing you can do when you know you are going to be giving test results is to suggest that patients bring a companion when they return for the result. This is sensible advice even if you do not yet know whether the results are good or bad. Another important consideration is to ensure that there is sufficient time for the consultation. When patients do bring companions with them, you will need to elicit and respond to everyone's questions and concerns. Avoid interruptions, and if possible ask someone to carry your bleep. Privacy is also very important to patients (Jurkovich *et al.*, 2000), so find a suitably private environment.

When you deliver bad news, in effect you are always going to be doing so on behalf of the team within which you work. Evidence suggests that junior doctors often do not have time to prepare themselves and are lacking support from other healthcare professionals; therefore, you should strive to prepare yourself and involve other team members (Dosanjh *et al.*, 2001). Consider how the other healthcare professionals on your team can help, because their support will be crucial for both you and the patient. Ask another member of the team, or a nurse or therapist who has been working closely with the patient, to accompany you.

During the consultation

Every patient is an individual, and so there is no 'right way' to break bad news. Unless you know the patient very well, it helps to start by finding out what they know already, what their understanding of the situation is, and what they are expecting from the consultation. This will help you give the news more gently if they have unrealistically optimistic expectations, but avoid an unnecessary preamble if they are fully prepared.

When delivering the news, be honest but try not to be too blunt. Try to ensure that the patient knows there is some difficult news coming, or that there is a possibility they will be disappointed, by giving them a 'warning shot', such as: **'It's not as simple as we first thought'** or just, **'It's not good news.'** This warning shot will increase their anxiety, but without it, the patient may be caught entirely unawares. Remember that patients will be exquisitely sensitive to these kinds of phrases, so it is important to follow with a full and clear explanation. It is also important to leave space for

A PATIENT'S PERSPECTIVE ON RECEIVING BAD NEWS

John Diamond was a journalist who died of cancer, and wrote wittily and movingly about his illness. Here is a short extract from his book *Snake Oil and Other Preoccupations* (Diamond, 2001) in which he talks about his experience with oncologists:

"What doctors need to know is how to bridge that two-second gap between opening the door of the room in which your terrified patient is waiting with his wife and speaking the first words. What do you do? Downcast eyes? Affected jollity? Thin, sympathetic smile? Pretend to be flicking through your notes as if they might have changed since you last looked at them? Maintain a chatty conversation with the accompanying nurse then turn to the patient – rather as those afternoon television hosts pretend to be engrossed in conversation until they notice the camera is on them?

Believe me, I've had them all. And the best is my oncologist. I mean it. He'd just given me the news the other day and I found that the only thing I could write down in response was 'God, but you did that so well.' Which sounds sarcastic, but it absolutely isn't intended as such. After all, as I told you the other week, I was pretty certain what the news would be. We sat in the room, and the door swung open and he looked straight at me with no artfully composed face, and said 'We're going to have to start treatment again,' as he walked in and sat down.

No messing. And especially no, 'How are you then?' Why do doctors ask that? They've got the damned case-notes in front of them and they know how you are with rather more accuracy than you do. Sometimes they vary this: 'How are you feeling then?' to which the only answer is, 'Tell me whether the cancer's back and I'll tell you how I'm feeling."

Diamond (2001)

realistic hope without making promises you cannot keep.

Evidence suggests that patients value both expertise and openness when bad news is being broken (Burkitt *et al.*, 2004; Hagerty *et al.*, 2005). Patients want their doctor to be up to date on the facts, but also to take time to answer questions completely, and to be honest about the severity of the situation (Parker *et al.*, 2001). Brusqueness, lack of sympathy, impatience, or inconsistencies can lead patients to view the doctor unfavourably (Barnett, 2002).

You will need to pace the delivery of information to suit the patient. If they are ready to hear a full explanation, then give it, remembering that people often need prompting to ask questions (Butow *et al.*, 1994). See below for advice on talking about prognosis. Conversely, some patients will need time for things to sink in before they are ready to move on to discussing details. You could ask them, **'Would you like to discuss the details of treatment now or leave it until another day?'** If appropriate, ask the patient, **'Is there anything you'd prefer not to be told?'** You may have to rely on non-verbal clues to tell you when to pause; watch the patient's face closely for signs that they are confused or feeling strong emotions. If they become very quiet, resist using the opportunity to talk about treatment options and so on, and wait until you think they are ready or until they ask a question before you move on. Silence may feel uncomfortable to you, but it can be very valuable.

Guidelines for breaking bad news often focus on the interaction between the doctor and the patient, and may neglect communication with patients' companions, even though over 90% of patients in one study brought someone else with them to the consultation (Eggly *et al.*, 2006). Difficulties may arise when the patient has heard enough, but their companion wants to ask questions, or vice versa. If this happens, acknowledge the difference in information requirements and find out whether the patient is happy for you to go on and answer the questions. Another possibility is to meet and talk with the companion separately, as long as you have the patient's explicit consent to do so. See Chapter 6 in this book for further discussion on this point.

Bear in mind that you cannot anticipate what the implications of the news will be for the patient. It may provoke a range of emotions – shock, anger, disbelief, denial, acceptance – or just an emotional blank. To ensure you have correctly read someone's emotional state, actively identify the emotion to yourself, for example, is it fear or anger? If you are unsure what the person is thinking or feeling, use an open question to find out. Once you have identified the emotion, clarify in your mind the specific reason for it. This may be obvious, but again, if you are not sure, ask. Finally, show that you have connected the emotion and the reason by saying something like, **'I can see that you're very shocked by what I've said.'** Try to be as specific as possible, rather than using a bland platitude. If the patient is tearful, it is usually appropriate to have a period of silence and possibly offer a tissue, but try to avoid giving the impression that they should 'pull themselves together'.

WHAT TO DO WHEN NOTHING YOU CAN SAY WILL MAKE THE SITUATION ANY BETTER

Sadly, there are some situations in medicine that are so terrible that nothing you can say will make the situation any better. For example, you may have to break the news of a sudden or unexpected death. In these cases, although you cannot make the situation any better, there is still much you can do to avoid making things worse and to help people come to terms with what has happened.

After you have followed the advice above on delivering the news in an honest but sensitive way, the next important thing to do is to stay with and support the patient and their companions. Try to avoid giving the impression that you are unconcerned about their emotions – don't change the subject, don't bring up practicalities too soon, don't suggest that their distress is normal, and don't try to cheer them up (Maguire & Pitceathly, 2002). A period of silence will usually be appropriate. Once you have given sufficient opportunity for the expression of emotions and you have an idea how the person is reacting, it will become clearer to you what to do next. Many people want privacy and solitude at these terrible times. There may also be practical concerns with which you can assist, such as producing the death certificate or phoning other relatives. If you knew the deceased, you may want to say something about them; for example, you could say how calm and dignified they were or reassure the relatives that the patient was not alone or in pain when they died.

After the consultation

After you have broken bad news, it is crucial to finish the consultation by making a clear plan for what will happen next. It may not be appropriate to formulate the treatment plan immediately. If you have just given the patient a new diagnosis, they may be too shocked to participate in decision making (Beaver *et al.*, 1996). Even if you are not making a full treatment plan, the patient should leave the consultation with a clear understanding about who to ask if they have more questions and what to do if things get worse. It should also be clear when you are going to meet again. The length of time needed between the first consultation and any subsequent meetings to discuss the treatment

WHAT TO SAY IF THE PATIENT ASKS 'HOW LONG HAVE I GOT TO LIVE?'

Doctors dread being asked this question. It is always difficult to answer accurately, and difficult to discuss without causing distress. However, if a patient asks you, then they usually have a good reason for doing so. It can also be a sign that they are coming to terms with their illness.

Try to find out why the patient wants to know, and what they really mean. For example, are they planning a family wedding or have they read something in the paper that has given them unrealistically good or bad expectations? Once you have understood the patient's perspective and you are sure they really want to have this discussion, consider carefully what to say. Firstly, make sure you know the median survival for patients with that diagnosis, to give yourself a 'ballpark' figure. One study found that doctors systematically overestimated survival times by a factor of up to five (Christakis & Lamont, 2000). Admit to the patient that you do not know exactly how long they will live, and that no one knows. Then give an answer that does not include a number. For example, if the median survival is 6 months, you might say, **'Months rather than years.'** You could also talk about fixed time points or events, especially if the patient has indicated that this is a concern. For example, if a patient mentions that they have a family wedding planned for some time in the distant future, you could say, **'I'm really sorry to have to say this, but I think you might want to consider bringing the wedding forward, as you may be too unwell by that time.'**

If you think the patient might die very soon, it is very important to try to convey this. For example, you could say, **'I think it won't be long. It could even happen in the next few days.'** It can also be helpful to discuss anything important that the patient wants to do before they die and whether you can help in practical ways to facilitate this. There are more or less explicit ways of asking this question, depending on the patient. For example: **'Is there anything you can do that will help give you peace of mind?'** Or **'Of all the things you would like to do, can you think of the most important to you?'**

plan may be very short, and should be guided by the patient if possible.

After the consultation, relay the results of the discussion to the rest of your team, write it in the patient's notes, and if possible tell the patient's GP. This allows for continuity of care, and will help to ensure that patients receive appropriate communication and support from the other healthcare professionals. There is evidence that patients do not accept bad news the first time it is told to them, so it is very likely that follow-up consultations with other members of the team, the nursing staff, or the patient's GP will be necessary (Wittenberg-Lyles *et al.*, 2008). At this point, you should also consider whether to arrange support for the patient from a clinical nurse specialist, a counsellor, a social worker, the palliative care team, or from the patient's friends and relatives.

Coping strategies to deal with the aftermath when another professional has broken bad news

While you are still a student, it may happen that a patient asks you to clarify statements made by senior doctors, especially after they have experienced a complex or upsetting consultation. If this happens to you, the first thing to do is listen carefully to the patient and show empathy with them. Explain that you are a student, and say that you can see that the patient is concerned and that their questions need to be addressed by one of the doctors. Then arrange for a qualified member of the team to speak with the patient. Do not attempt to answer the patient's questions yourself, even if you feel you know the answers, as you may find yourself launching unawares into a complex discussion of prognosis or end of life.

A common situation for junior doctors is that a patient or relative asks a question about some bad news that has already been broken by someone else. For example, a patient might catch you after the ward round, and ask, **'Can you just explain what Dr Smith meant when he said the cancer is in my lungs? Have I got lung cancer?'** In this situation, you will need to follow the procedure for breaking bad news, even though you may feel that the news has already been broken. You will not just be clarifying terminology or comforting the patient, you will be performing an essential role in helping them to understand and come to terms with the information they have been given.

When you *are* a junior doctor, if a patient or relative asks to speak to you after they have been told bad news, you will usually need to do some preparation. Tell the patient you will come back in 10 minutes, and then go and acquaint yourself with the medical details

and try to find out what they have already been told. Ensure you have enough time and you are in the right frame of mind before you start the consultation. Begin by clarifying what the patient understands. You could say something like, **'What did you understand about your condition from the other doctor?'** Patients may have misunderstood, may recall very little of what was said, or may choose to say they cannot remember, in the hope that there has been some kind of mistake. In these cases, you will need to go back gently and recap the previous conversation, answering any additional questions the patient has, while avoiding introducing any inconsistencies.

These 'aftermath' consultations can be very challenging. You cannot possibly know in advance whether the patient simply needs a listening ear, whether they have seriously misunderstood the situation, whether they have multiple questions that need answering, or all three. Either way, you are playing an essential role in helping the patient come to terms with the situation they are facing.

Talking to patients who are in pain or dying

Talking to patients who are extremely ill or in pain can be very difficult. Students usually stay away from such situations to avoid causing unnecessary distress. However, as a newly qualified doctor it will be a necessary and frequent part of your work, and one for which you may find yourself poorly prepared. The best training you can get is to accompany the palliative care team on their rounds and learn from their behaviour. There are many practical things you can do to maintain patients' dignity and comfort towards the end of life.

When you go in to see an extremely ill patient, remind yourself how you feel when you are very ill or in severe pain. Assume the patient is aware of you and talk to them in a normal or quiet voice, even if they appear unconscious or semi-conscious. Introduce yourself carefully, especially if they have their eyes shut. Ask permission before touching or examining them, and watch their face closely. Even very weak or semi-conscious patients may be able to respond to you by blinking, nodding, or squeezing your hand. Look carefully for any signs of distress, including grimaces, restlessness, confused speech or noises, and tachycardia or tachypnoea. Avoid any unnecessary interventions, but conversely do not just rush in and out of the room; spend some time with them, even if it is in silence. Consider whether there is anything you can do to improve the patient's comfort. Communication with the patient's loved ones becomes very important at this time, so remember to ask them whether they have any requests.

Dealing with your own emotions

After breaking bad news, you are likely to feel terrible. Studies have shown that doctors experience a wide range of negative emotions after breaking bad news, including fear that the patient will think badly of them, guilt, sadness, anxiety, and a strong sense of responsibility for the situation (Fallowfield & Jenkins, 2004; Tesser *et al.*, 1971). Remind yourself that you are not responsible for the bad news, only for conveying that information to the patient. If you feel very upset, take some time to yourself, or talk to a colleague, a friend, or your partner. Don't just carry on as if nothing has happened – remember that these consultations are probably the hardest part of your job.

Having a good working relationship with the other healthcare professionals in your team will help. When you need to break bad news, ask a colleague to accompany you. This has advantages both for the patient and for you. After the consultation, you can ask your colleague for feedback and talk through what happened. Colleagues will respect you for your openness and humility, and are much more likely to give you praise than criticism. Any feedback you receive will help you develop your communication skills and become better at your job. A debrief can be especially helpful if the patient has had an extreme reaction to the news. If repeated consultations will be necessary over a period of time, try to get the same colleague to 'buddy' you for each consultation.

You may find that there are times when your personal life affects your ability to cope with these difficult consultations. If you have had a recent loss or bereavement, or if you are going through a difficult time at home, you may become more than usually emotional. If possible, you should try to avoid crying in front of patients, as this can convey a message of hopelessness (Friedrichsen *et al.*, 2000). If you do cry, it may help to acknowledge it by saying something like, **'Your situation is very difficult; it's upset me too.'** If you are feeling particularly vulnerable for some reason, then try to get support from other members of your multidisciplinary team. Most healthcare professionals will have been in similar situations themselves at some point, so they will understand. It may be possible to ask someone else to break the bad news for you, so long as it will not be detrimental to the patient's care.

Summary

As a student, you still have a part to play in supporting patients and relatives to come to terms with bad news, even though it has been broken by another healthcare professional. As a junior doctor, remember that whenever you are giving information to a patient or their relative, you are potentially breaking bad news. When you do so, follow the advice in this chapter: prepare yourself, find out as much as you can about the medical details and what the patient has already been told, and take your time when you do talk to the patient. Remember your own needs, and consider the effect such consultations may have on you. Think through the strategies and support you have or will need to help you cope.

Further reading

Baile, W., Buckman, R., Lenzi, R., Glober, G., Beale, E., and Kudelka, A. (2000). SPIKES – A six-step protocol for delivering bad news: Application to the patient with cancer. *The Oncologist* **5**(4), 302–311.

Fallowfield, L. and Jenkins, V. (2004). Communicating sad, bad, and difficult news in medicine. *The Lancet*, **363**(9405), 312–319.

Macdonald, E. (Ed.) (2004). *Difficult Conversations in Medicine*. Oxford: Oxford University Press.

Visit the Online Resource Centre for *Clinical Communication Skills* at: www.oxfordtextbooks.co.uk/orc/washer

References

Barnett, M. (2002). Effect of breaking bad news on patients' perceptions of doctors. *Journal of the Royal Society of Medicine*, **95**(7), 343–347.

Beaver, K., Luker, K.A., Owens, R.G., Leinster, S.J., Degner, L.F., and Sloan, J.A. (1996). Treatment decision making in women newly diagnosed with breast cancer. *Cancer Nursing*, **19**(1), 8–19.

Burkitt Wright, E., Holcombe, C., and Salmon, P. (2004). Doctors' communication of trust, care, and respect in breast cancer: Qualitative study. *British Medical Journal*, **328**(7444), 864–868.

Butow, P.N., Dunn, S.M., Tattersall, M.H.N., and Jones, Q.J. (1994). Patient participation in the cancer consultation; Evaluation of a question prompt sheet. *Annals of Oncology*, **5**(3), 199–204.

Christakis, N. and Lamont, E. (2000). Extent and determinants of error in doctors' prognoses in terminally ill patients: Prospective cohort study. *British Medical Journal*, **320**(7233), 469–473.

Diamond, J. (2001). *Snake Oil and Other Preoccupations*. London: Vintage.

Dosanjh, S., Barnes, J., and Bhandari, M. (2001). Barriers to breaking bad news among medical and surgical residents. *Medical Education*, **35**(3), 197–205.

Eggly, S., Penner, L., Albrecht, T., Cline, R., Foster, T., Naughton, M., Peterson, A., and Ruckdeschel, J. (2006). Discussing bad news in the outpatient oncology clinic: Rethinking current communication guidelines. *Journal of Clinical Oncology*, **24**(4), 716–719.

Fallowfield, L. and Jenkins, V. (2004). Communicating sad, bad, and difficult news in medicine. *The Lancet*, **363**(9405), 312–319.

Friedrichsen, M., Strang, P., and Carlsson, M. (2000). Breaking bad news in the transition from curative to palliative cancer care – Patient's view of the doctor giving the information. *Support Care Cancer*, **8**(6), 472–478.

Hagerty, R., Butow, P.N., Ellis, P.M., Lobb, E., Pendlebury, S., Leigh, N., MacLeod, C., and Tattersall, M.H. (2005). Communicating with realism and hope: Incurable cancer patients' views on the disclosure of prognosis. *Journal of Clinical Oncology*, **23**(6), 1278–1288.

Jenkins, V., Fallowfield, L., and Saul, J. (2001). Information needs of patients with cancer: Results from a large study in UK cancer centres. *British Journal of Cancer*, **84**(1), 48–51.

Jurkovich, G., Pierce, B., Pananen, L., and Rivara, F. (2000). Giving bad news: The family perspective. *Journal of Trauma*, **48**(5), 865–870.

Maguire, P. and Pitceathly, C. (2002). Key communication skills and how to acquire them. *British Medical Journal*, **325**(7366), 697–700.

Parker, P., Baile, W.F., de Moor, C., Lenzi, R., Kudelka, A.P., and Cohen, L. (2001). Breaking bad news about cancer: Patients' preferences for communication. *Journal of Clinical Oncology*, **19**(7), 2049–2056.

Schildmann, J., Cushing, A., Doyal, L., and Vollmann, J. (2005). Breaking bad news: Experiences, views and difficulties of pre-registration house officers. *Palliative Medicine*, **19**(2), 93–98.

Tesser, A., Rosen, S., and Tesser, M. (1971). On the reluctance to communicate undesirable messages (the MUM effect). A field study. *Psychological Reports*, **29**, 651–654.

Wittenberg-Lyles, E., Goldsmith, J., Sanchez-Reilly, S., and Ragan, S. (2008). Communicating a terminal prognosis in a palliative care setting: Deficiencies in current communication training protocols. *Social Science and Medicine*, **66**, 2356–2365.

How to do well in communication skills OSCEs

Peter Washer

This book has hopefully helped you learn how to communicate in a variety of contexts with patients, their families, and with other professionals. One more thing that you will need to learn how to do is to demonstrate what you have learned in assessments. You will be assessed on your communication skills throughout your career. As a student, your communication skills, as well as other aspects of your clinical competence, are usually assessed through Objective Structured Clinical Examinations (OSCEs).

OSCEs are a standardized examination in which each candidate moves through a series of 'stations' designed to test different aspects of your clinical and communication skills. The communication skills stations tend to have simulated patients (actors) who will each have an outline of a script of their character, although they will respond to how empathic (or not) each candidate is. The pressure of OSCEs, particularly at final examinations, is intense, and they are often dreaded by students. This final section aims to give you some practical tips to help you do your best in OSCEs, and is based on my own experience in setting communication skills OSCEs, training OSCE examiners, and examining many hundreds of candidates in OSCEs over the years.

I hope this advice, and indeed the advice given throughout this book, will be useful to you. I wish you well in your exams and in your careers. You have chosen wisely – medicine is one of the most rewarding careers there is. Remember that working with patients and their families is truly a privilege – and enjoy it.

TIPS ON DOING WELL IN COMMUNICATION SKILLS OSCES

- As in any examination, read and re-read the question or the station instructions carefully.

- Make a mental plan of what you are going to cover, or write some bullet points on a scrap of paper, before you start talking.

- Remember to introduce yourself properly. Nervous candidates are often so eager to get on to the content of the interview that they forget to say who they are or check the patient's name. There will usually be marks for your introduction. These marks are easily gained – and lost.

- Do not be afraid to rearrange the chairs if you feel it would be beneficial.

- The simulated patient will have an outline of a script and they will tell you everything you need to know – if you let them! Start with an open question and do not interrupt the simulated patient while they are telling you the problem.

- The OSCE is primarily an opportunity for you to show that you can empathize and respond to patients – your clinical knowledge can be tested elsewhere. Some students seem to think, for example, that a station where the simulated patient is asking for smoking cessation advice is an opportunity for them to show off that they have learned all the latest nicotine replacement therapies. Those students will do less well than those who explore what smoking *means* to this person, who empathize with how difficult it is to stop, *and* offer the latest nicotine replacement advice.

- You usually get a warning bell or announcement a few minutes before you need to move to the next station – this warning bell is your opportunity to start to wrap the interview up. You should not introduce new information at this stage, just summarize and check that the patient understands, and if they have any final concerns. If you have not covered everything you wanted to, say, 'If I can just summarize: we've talked about [a, b, and c], but we've run out of time, and we need to talk about [x, y, and z]. Why don't you make another appointment, and perhaps bring your partner along, and we can continue talking about the things we haven't had a chance to cover today?' This flags up to the examiner that you have run out of time, rather than forgotten to cover some of the material you should have.

- Remember that even if a station is not clearly a 'COMMUNICATION SKILLS' station, if there is a patient or a simulated patient in a station, there are likely to be marks allocated to your communication skills. Just because the instructions say 'Examine this patient and reach a diagnosis', rather than 'Explore this person's concerns', it doesn't mean that you can forget about introducing yourself, starting with an open question, being empathic, and so on. (See the summary list at the end of Chapter 2.)

- Simulated patients are often briefed to give you cues and clues. Look out for these and respond to them. So, for example, if a simulated patient says 'I was feeling worried . . .' respond with, 'Was there anything in particular you were worried about?' This is not rocket science, but you would be amazed at how, under examination conditions, students and even experienced doctors let obvious cues and clues sail by without acknowledging or responding to them because they are so busy concentrating on the clinical detail or the task in hand.

- The examiner's role is to check your name and candidate number and usually to observe your performance without interaction. Sometimes the examiner's role is also to ask a specific question(s), which will be the same questions asked to all students. Do not ask the examiner for feedback on how you have done at the end of the station, as they will not be able to tell you either way.

Transcript of Alice's podcast

Go to www.oxfordtextbooks.co.uk/orc/washer/ to listen to the audio recording of this interview.

'Hello. I'm Peter Washer the editor of Clinical Communication Skills and I am joined in this podcast by Alice. I'm in Alice's home, which is close to a railway track, so you might hear the trains rumbling by in the background. Welcome Alice, tell me about yourself.'

'I look after my partner who has had a number of strokes, he is quite severely disabled now, he gradually became more and more disabled, but he is quite severely disabled physically, also, slowly mentally as well, he is less able to concentrate and less able to hold a conversation. Also his speech is gradually been affected.'

'. . . And how long have you been caring for him?'

'For the past 9 years.'

'So in that 9 years you would have had quite a lot of experience of doctors and their communication skills?'

'Yes quite a lot.'

'Tell me your thoughts.'

'Well we've had problems with trying to understand what the doctors would say and feeling very rushed, when we went in the hospital where the staff have very limited time to spare.'

'When you say you've had problem understanding what the doctors were saying, what exactly do you mean by that?'

'Well, basically because they use their own jargon most of the time, this really for an everyday person it means nothing.'

'So if a doctor were to use some sort of medical jargon or a medical concept you didn't understand, would you not just feel able to ask them to explain it to you?'

'Yes of course I would. Sometimes I try to work it out in my head and try to make sense of what they are saying, thinking that I may be able to understand at the end of it what they were actually saying. But some other times they may use very technical terms, terms I really wouldn't understand, and if I repeat it, if I ask them to repeat it they may repeat the same thing.'

'Right, so can you give me an example?'

'Well recently my partner fell ill and I was worried about the symptoms that he was showing, because he had pancreatitis before – I didn't know whether it was a repeat of the pancreatitis, or problems with the liver, or even problems with anaemia.'

'. . . And how did the doctor explain that to you?'

'When I asked her if she had the results of the blood tests, she, regarding the pancreas, she gave the count of I expect the enzymes, which meant nothing to me. She said the count was better and she gave the count as opposed to the previous one but it did not mean anything to me.'

'So what did you want to hear?'

'I wanted to hear of course giving me the count of the enzyme count, if that was the problem, but to tell me that it was either better or it was an improvement, she could have just said in simple words, 'There was problem with the pancreas, but it has got better now', and if I wanted more explanation then I could have asked her.'

'. . . So perhaps to start more simply first.'

'Simply first, and then if someone is knowledgeable in this field then of course they would have asked more questions.'

'Of course. And when were talking earlier you said that your partner was in hospital recently and so he's been to two different accident and emergency departments recently and you said there was a contrast between those two, do you want to tell me about that?'

'Yes, within a couple of weeks we went into two different hospitals. The first hospital was extremely busy, we didn't really have any explanation of what was happening or what they were doing and we spent quite a number of hours there, really without proper information as to what they were doing there basically. I still didn't know what was wrong with him. The second hospital we went to was very different in that they were less rushed, perhaps was a less busy time or perhaps a less busy hospital altogether in the A&E, but it was less rushed and whether it was and a nurse or a doctor, somebody came every half hour or every hour to tell us what they were going to do next, which was all we needed, and then you feel more at ease and less pressured.'

'So it sounds like the issue is not that you were kept waiting because you were obviously you are prepared for that, but that you were kept waiting without being given explanations of what was going on and that was really important for you?'

'Yes exactly. Waiting in A&E or at any time in hospital is something we expect in a sense. But waiting without being told what is going to happen makes it far more stressful, we are already under pressure especially when somebody has been suddenly taken to hospital because they are very ill, then we already are under a great deal of pressure and stress and therefore we need to have feedback and to be put at ease that things are going to be done.'

'Ok, thank you very much Alice for that, that's been really helpful, thank you.'

'Thank you very much.'

Transcript of Casey's podcast

Go to www.oxfordtextbooks.co.uk/orc/washer/ to listen to the audio recording of this interview.

'Hello I'm Peter Washer the editor of Clinical Communication Skills, and in this podcast I am joined by Dr Caroline Fertleman who is a consultant paediatrician at the Whittington hospital in North London, and by Casey, who is a patient here at the Whittington. Welcome both.'

'Tell me Casey, tell me something about yourself.'

'My name is Casey, I am thirteen years old, I used to have leukaemia – it went on for three and half years.'

'So when were you diagnosed with leukaemia?'

'When I was seven years old and I'm now thirteen.'

'So tell me something about what was like to have had leukaemia when you were seven, for the three years.'

'Horrible, because I felt that I was different, I thought I felt very different because when I lost my hair some people would take the mick' [make fun of] and I was bullied in primary school for it and that wasn't very nice.'

'And were you in hospital for a long period?'

'Yeah.'

'How long?'

'Three and half years, and if I am at home you never knew if I'd have to be rushed back to the hospital, and I did not know if the day would be my last day, I didn't know if I would pass away that day.'

'You must have had a really tough time. As you know this podcast is for a book about communication skills for medical students. So tell me what your experiences of doctor's communication skills have been like?'

'Doctors are actually good because they talk, they understand, they understand my point of view, yeah that was just nice.'

'Can you tell me more about what you thought was good about them?'

'If I needed to have injections they would do it on my count. Like if I said, 'Can you do it on 3?', and then I would count to three and then they'll do it.'

'So one of the things that is really good from your point of view was that they would let you know if you were going to have treatment in advance so it wouldn't sort of surprise you with it. What about explaining things to you, were they good at that?'

'They did explain a lot of these things me, that's how I would like it, I liked to be kept in the loop, to know what was going on.'

'Did they explain about your medicines and what the side effects were? You don't have to remember all the medicines because it was a long time ago now, but do you remember what side effects were and did they explain them to you?'

'I can't really remember the side effects, but I do know that there were a lot of side effects, and one of them was that I lost control of my legs and couldn't walk for a little while.'

'That must have been really, really scary, how did they explain that to you?'

'They said to me that I would hopefully get my legs back working and stuff like that, and I believed that because I just tried to keep positive.'

'This must have been not only hard on you but hard on your mum as well. Your mum would have been around hospital with you a lot. How do you feel when the doctors were talking to you when your mum was there and did you feel they were talking to you or to your mum, did they get it right or was there something you would like them to have done differently?'

'I didn't like to be woken up in the middle of the night. Every day was hard for me been awaken. Most of the time when I was in hospital I wasn't allowed out of my room because of infections, and having no antibodies and stuff like that. I did not like be woken up at night, because I would be very tired. I remember when I used to be woken up in the night I used to hit the nurses by accident because of stuff like that.'

'What about, Peter asked you a question about your mum, did you feel the doctors talked to you or did they talk up to you, did they patronise you, or did they talk to your mum then your mum explain things to you, how did it usually work?'

'Sometimes they would talk to both of us at the same time but some times they would call my mum away, talk to my mum and then my mum would talk to me. So like it was a mixture, but most of the time they would talk to my mum and then my mum would tell me. I wasn't upset with that because I was getting told anyway.'

'Did you ever get upset about this? Having leukaemia is obviously an upsetting time how did if you and your mum were upset, what would happen?'

'I saw it as – I was upset, who wouldn't be? But I had it, it wasn't going to go away that day. There is no point getting upset, I just had to get on with it, wait for today because now I am happy with my life and life is better.'

'Good, that is a really nice positive note to end on. Before we finish, is there anything that you particularly, this is going to be listened by medical students, is there anything, a take home message? What sort of things you would like it be when they talk to children?'

'When they talk to children? Try and be honest with them, because that is what children like, honesty. Yeah, to be honest.'

'Thanks very much Casey.'

'That was brilliant, that was really good actually.'

Transcript of Catherine's podcast

Go to www.oxfordtextbooks.co.uk/orc/washer/ to listen to the audio recording of this interview.

'Hello. My name is Peter Washer and I am the editor of Clinical Communication Skills. I am joined in this podcast by Mrs Catherine Webster. Catherine tell me something about yourself.'

'My husband and I have been married for fifty years, and we have 3 children and the second child who was born in 1964 clearly had all sorts of physical problems and was in hospital for 8 months, but we did not have a diagnosis until she was 4 and a half.'

'And the diagnosis when you got it was?'

'Prader-Willi Syndrome.'

'Prader-Willi Syndrome. And how is that affect your daughter?'

'Well it affects children in very complicated ways, but the chief, the two chief areas of the brain damage, the deletion of chromosome 15 are hyperphasia, feeling, thinking about food the whole time, akin feeling of starvation, there is not feeling of satiety. So this affects daily life in an extreme way, and the other main one I'd say is temper control which is also affected. So affable nice children, when they get upset, they get terribly upset.'

'So over the years you would have had a lot of experience of doctor's communication skills, in general what has been your impression?'

'In general we've been extremely fortunate. We did have one bad experience over the diagnosis. That doctor had worked with doctors Prader, Willi and Laphart, and he was so excited to find a child with this. It was patent he was so excited, it didn't make me feel he was thinking about the child or us as a family. And I'm afraid we found out later he'd give her blood tests

which she didn't need to have, which was very sad. But that is the outstanding bad negative experience, the rest have been just as good.'

'So what, let's focus on the good ones, if they kind of outweighed the bad ones, what has made them good.'

'They were wonderful human beings I think and they focused on our daughter and us as a family, me, and they gave us very helpful support. Even if it meant, with the weight control when it went gradually out of control, even it meant frightening us as a consequence, but that was helpful too.'

'Can I just go back to this question of them being wonderful human beings, how do you know they were wonderful human beings, can we teach that to medical students?'

'You can I am sure you can, yes. [laughs] Well, concrete example perhaps, when the professor at Great Ormond Street, [children's hospital] when we came into the room he would exclaim our daughter's name with such enthusiasm, as if she was the one person he most wanted to see, and he focused on her first.'

'And that helped you as well?'

'Of course.'

'And presumably this, having middle siblings a middle child of three with this condition is going to put a lot of strain on the whole family?'

'Yes indeed it does.'

'How can doctors help there?'

'I think that must be pointed out, that attention and to make sure the family knows that they know they must give attention to the other children and . . .'

'. . . both parents . . .'

'. . . and to both parents. Yes the emphasis on looking after the father, I think. I was taught by one friend who is an endocrinologist, who said looking after the fathers, it's so important.'

'You were telling me earlier that one of the other things that you really valued about doctors' communication skills was when they are not afraid to tackle difficult issues with you.'

'Thats right, yes. Yes, that was particularly so. This condition means it's almost impossible for boys to have children and for girls to have children and this is something that most of the people with Prader-Willi Syndrome long to have. They are very affectionate, and our daughter wanted to talk about that I know, but it was the one thing I had a hang up about. I could talk to her about all sorts of things, but not about sex and having babies, but the professor said to me, 'You know I find in my work that', especially when he said he went to talk to children that are terminally ill, 'the one subject they most wanted to talk about and that everybody tended to avoid was their condition, that they were going to die, and how they were going to die'. So he related that to my hesitancy in talking about sex and having babies.'

'. . . and as a result of that conversation with the professor you were able to go and have that conversation with your daughter?'

'Yes, which she took very well I must say, she knew about sex, she told me 'Oh we've done that in school', but it was the issue of having babies.'

'Thanks very much for that Mrs Webster, that's been really useful, thank you.'

Transcript of Eileen's podcast

Go to www.oxfordtextbooks.co.uk/orc/washer/ to listen to the audio recording of this interview.

'Hello I am Peter Washer and I am the editor of Clinical Communication Skills and I am joined in this podcast by Dr Eileen Rosenfelder, Eileen tell me about yourself.'

'Hi there, I am a GP and I qualified at University College Hospital in 1985, and before becoming a GP spent some time in paediatrics as well. I work in medical education and wanted to share some of my thoughts on time efficiency with the students, because that's going to be the big thing that it is going to hit you when you qualify.'

'OK, you are very busy as a GP, you've got a big waiting room full of people and how do you manage that? How do you steer a course between not appearing rushed and between making sure that they all get their slot?'

'The first thing to do is to compose yourself in between each patient and always try to have looked at the patient's records before you called them in. It may be just to look at the drugs in the computer when they were last seen and maybe a quick summary. In our practice we still have A4 folders still and I will leaf through and try to make sure I have a good grip, particularly on their drug history before they come in.'

'So preparation before they actually walk through the door?'

'Definitely, it is always worth it and you think it is slowing you down but actually it's saving a lot of time and make you a lot safer. When I called the patient in I always, always start with an open question, I'll say, I introduce myself if they haven't met me and I say 'Please sit down', and then I usually start with 'How can I help?' In general start with an open question, and one of the most useful tips I would say is let the patient speak uninterrupted for a good one to two minutes, even you are feeling the pressure of the full waiting room and the time, the clock ticking. Just wait let them speak, because they will usually reveal a lot if you don't interrupt them and then you can actually ask the closed more pertinent questions that you have much more efficiently. If you interrupt too early on, the patient will forget what they have come with and they'll remember later in the conversation and it actually makes you much more inefficient. The other useful tip is if the patient comes and says, 'I've got a long list of things for you doctor', you say, 'That's fine, just run how many points there are on your list and then I'll say will see how much time we have for today'. Be advised that the thing that they really worried about will be often at the end of the list. I had a lady the other day who came and show a rash on her back and then she said, 'Could I . . . ?, she wanted to talk about her bowels, she had a bit of diarrhoea, and then she said, 'There's just one other thing' and then she started to tell me about her central chest pain that developed over the last three weeks, and as ever she left the thing that was really worrying her to the last minute, the last point.'

'OK, I am also interested in what your thoughts are as they are learning all these skills, how to take history, how to give information and so on in communication skills but when they come to be doctors they need to do that a lot quicker, what sort of message have you got about, around that?'

'You'll find once you qualify you will see a lot more patients that you become much quicker at taking histories because you are not struggling around to think what is the next question, it just flows much more naturally. The most important thing I would say is don't appear rushed to the patient. An agitated doctor who's checking their watch or looking at the clock the whole time or who appears distracted will put the patient off. Once the patient has been put off you they will lose confidence in you'll have to struggle hard to regain that confidence, if you are in fact successful. You in fact may be very bright and very capable, but when a colleague comes along their patients will soon tell them, 'Oh I didn't like that doctor, they didn't seem to have any time for me at all'. I can give you a useful example here, particularly as I emphasised earlier about taking good drug histories in your preparation. I saw a patient the other day who had bruising under his skin and I knew he was on Warfarin and I said, 'What's going on?' and he'd been given antibiotics for what appeared to be a simple chest infection by a colleague and I said, 'Well didn't he tell you to go and get your INR checked?' and the patient told me at the start he had only two minutes for me and it was going to be a quick check of his chest. So obviously that was an example of bad medicine. You've always, always, always got to check the drug histories, you've always got to stop and think; what am I missing? Even if you just got two to three minutes, you must compose yourself, you must think clearly. Before you give a prescription you must always check what drugs interactions could occur, what allergies does this patient have, and if I would give one teaching message I would say that. I remember when I was a medical student the professor of pharmacology saying to us. 'If you forget to ask a patient if they are allergic to penicillin that is really negligent', and that has always stayed with me: that there are some bottom lines as a doctor that you just cannot afford to miss, and I hope looking back over my career I have always asked that question. I think I have.'

'OK great that is really useful Eileen, thanks very much.'

Transcript of Kitty's podcast

Go to www.oxfordtextbooks.co.uk/orc/washer/ to listen to the audio recording of this interview.

'Hello, my name is Peter Washer and I am the editor of Clinical Communication Skills and I'm joined in this podcast by Dr Kitty Mohan, Kitty tell me about yourself.'

'My name is Kitty and I qualified about three and half years ago from medical school and I am currently working as a doctor.'

'OK, so you would have been one of the first generation, given when you qualified you would have been one of the first generation, to go through the new medical curriculum where you were formally taught communication skills, as opposed to previous generations of doctors who would have learnt it as part of the apprenticeship. Tell me about that, how was it for you as a medical student learning communication skills?'

'It was quite an interesting experience being taught how to communicate, because you presume you know how to communicate. I think at that time I found that it was fun, that it was quite enjoyable, I quite enjoyed the scenarios, but I wasn't really sure how this was going to improve my practice when I qualified or how this was really very relevant.'

'OK, I mean were you an enthusiastic communication skills student, were you one of the people who volunteered for stuff?'

'Yes, [laughs] I was one of the people who always volunteered, I could not bear the idea of not.'

'OK, at the time they seemed quite fun and you were quite enthusiastic but it seem a bit unreal, is that it?'

'Yes.'

'So, three and half years ago you made this transition from being a medical student to being a doctor, I mean, how was that transition?'

'It was a really hard transition, I think that you are just not prepared for the idea. When you are a medical student you are now much more part of a team, but when you are doctor suddenly you're the person that has to make decisions, deal with the relatives and not just the actors and people like that.'

'So, did you feel that the communication skills that you'd learnt as a medical student was that useful when you became a doctor?'

'Yes, I think that it suddenly became very evident why we were taught communication skills. I think that when it is the middle of the night and you haven't slept for many hours you're on auto-pilot and you have actually at that stage rely on the skills that are really deeply embedded in your brain and you've being taught. It comes as second nature to you, and you are suddenly thankful really.'

'OK, that is a really positive message isn't it, because things that seem quite unreal at the time do provide you with some sort of resources, some sort of toolkit, and they are deeply embedded, as you say, that when you need to use them they're there.'

'Yeah.'

'And, do you notice a difference? I said that you're one of the first generation of doctors to have been formally taught communication skills in the way that we do now. Do you notice any difference between your generation of doctors and the previous generation that haven't been taught communication skills?'

'I think that's one of the most kind of surprising things, that I did actually notice a difference. I think the fact that you take it for granted that everyone's going to have a very set level of communication skills, but I think before people were taught it was very hit and miss what did they actually pick up. So I think you do notice that either the previous generation of doctors, or people who didn't train where they were formally taught communication skills, you realise that they don't actually have the same equipment and toolkit, as you put it, to rely on.'

'OK, that is a really useful message, thank you for that.'

'Thank you.'

Transcript of Megan's podcast

Go to www.oxfordtextbooks.co.uk/orc/washer/ to listen to the audio recording of this interview.

'Hello, my name is Peter Washer and I am the editor of Clinical Communication Skills, and in this podcast I am joined by Dr Caroline Fertleman, who is a consultant paediatrician at the Whittington Hospital in north London, and by Miss Megan Clifford who is going to talk about her experiences as a patient. So Megan, tell me something about yourself.'

'Ok, well, obviously my name is Megan Clifford, I am seventeen I'm studying health and social care at City and Islington College.'

'Tell us why you were in hospital.'

'I was in hospital with pneumonia on two occasions. Once when I was fourteen for about a week and then when I was sixteen for about three weeks. But when I was in hospital when I was sixteen with pneumonia I lost a lot of weight, I mean, I was down to 5 and a half stones, so you can imagine what I looked like. And suspicions, people thought I had an eating disorder because they caught me throwing away food as well.'

'Alright, so they caught you throwing away food, you can understand why they would think that. What was going on for you? '

'I mean, I know myself that I wasn't making myself sick, and I knew that I wasn't ill in that department and I thought there's a reason for why I'm not putting on weight and if you keep telling me I am anorexic we're not going to get to the bottom of this. You can't just say someone is ill.'

'So why were you throwing away food?'

'Generally because I didn't like it. I mean, it was a Build Up milkshake they had given me and they said it was really nice. I don't really like milk and dairy stuff as it is, and when I took a mouthful I thought, this is disgusting, and because I was in my own room I thought no-one was looking so I threw it away. As I was throwing it away the nurse walked in and she was like, 'I'm going to record this'. I can obviously understand why, I mean, they caught me throwing away a milkshake and mash potato on two separate occasions and that's when the doctors started saying that, 'Okay we think that you have an eating disorder, you are getting a bit ill and what not'.'

'As you know we're making this recording about how doctors talk to young people and children, tell us what have been your experiences? Maybe starting with the good and then move on to what could be better.'

'Well, like I said, when I was in the hospital with pneumonia the good part was when the doctor was telling me how ill I was. I mean to a stroppy sixteen-year old you just tell them they've got pneumonia they just think nothing, that it would be gone by next week. I didn't actually understand how ill I was until one day I said, 'I'm not listening to this and I am going out for a cigarette'. The doctor actually shouted a me and said, 'You can't go out for a cigarette, you don't understand how ill you are', and he sat me down and told me how ill I was. That was when I took a step back and I thought, okay I have got to start getting better now. It is not all about going outside to have a fag [cigarette] you know.'

'That doesn't sound very positive, being shouted at.'

'I mean I had to, someone had to shout at me, to tell me, because I was just not listening, after about two weeks the doctor was just getting a bit annoyed with me because I wasn't listening and then he was like, 'Do you know what Megan, you are very ill and you can't be going out for cigarettes all the time'.'

'Right, and nobody told you that before?'

'People don't like smokers anyway, so it was like, 'It's really bad for you, don't go out and smoke' and I was like, 'Whatever'. Then, I didn't know pneumonia was a lung infection, at that time I just thought, I didn't know what I thought, I was only young and that's when I was sat down and told it was a lung infection, you got bad asthma, you're on three inhalers, it's cold outside, you're only tiny, you've got to wrap up. That's when I thought, okay I am ill, that's what I thought was really good about it: that I am ill. That when they actually sat me down and told me that I am ill, and told me I couldn't do was I was doing.'

'And tell me when things weren't so good, you know when things happened when your mum was there?'

'The only thing I would say that wasn't very good was when the doctors they would prefer to talk to my mum, my parents, and wouldn't talk to me. I mean I was hard work, I admit that myself, I was very hard work, but I felt like that they couldn't talk to me, they had to talk to my mum and I was the third party you know. They'd tell my mum and then my mum would tell me, and I would tell my mum and she would tell the doctors. It just wasn't making a lot of sense to me. That is only thing I could say that was quite bad about the whole thing.'

'Right, so you would have preferred they had come directly to you?'

'Yeah.'

'With your mum there or without your mum there?'

'Maybe with my mum there, but talk to both if us because there were a few of occasions when I was asked to leave the room so they could speak to my mum and I thought, I'm not a little kid, I'm sixteen, they should tell me what's going on. That is the only thing I could say that was a bit bad in the whole thing and being told I was anorexic and that I had an eating disorder when I know I didn't.'

'What could they have done differently?'

'I mean they could have just tried to listen to me a bit more, because it was just like, 'You are anorexic, you are ill, you are not going home until you put on weight', and I thought I can't put on weight, I don't know why I am not putting on weight, I really do want to go home. And I thought to myself you just can't tell me I am anorexic because there's obviously something wrong with me if I'm not putting on weight and people need to get to the bottom of this because I've been in here twice with pneumonia and about my weight issues and I know myself that I don't make myself sick, I don't starve myself. Obviously to the doctors, catching me throwing away food they think differently.'

'So, have you got any take home messages, this is going to be listened by medical students, what sort of things would you like to say?'

'Don't undermine teenagers, don't think every teenager is just a stroppy teenager, because it's not like that. If you are in hospital unwell and you've been told you got an illness and you know you haven't got it. Just try to listen to them a little bit more, you know, because we are not all kids, some of us are very grown up and do we need to be heard sometimes.'

'Okay, thanks very much Megan.'

'That's okay.'

'Thank you Megan.'

Transcript of Michael's podcast

Go to www.oxfordtextbooks.co.uk/orc/washer/ to listen to the audio recording of this interview.

'Hello. My name is Peter Washer and in this podcast I am joined by Dr Michael Modell. Welcome Michael.'

'Hello.'

'Tell me about yourself.'

'Well, I am a retired professor of general practice from UCL [University College, London]. I entered medical school in 1955, and qualified in 1960. Then, after two years, went into general practice and I remained a partner in a north London general practice, with a very mixed clientele, for 30 years or so; combined general practice with academia, mainly teaching medical students, teaching medical students outside hospitals within the community, mainly in general practice. Then I left my practice in the 1990s and spent the remaining years of my professional career in academia.'

'So you were a medical student in the late 50s?'

'. . . in the late 50s.'

'So in those days how did you learn how to talk with your patients?'

'Well, there was no such thing as learning communication skills, I'm not sure if the phrase even existed at that time. We certainly amongst ourselves, amongst our fellow students, we talked, 'How do you talk to patients? How do you get them to tell you what is wrong with them? How do you put them at your ease? And that was a quite an important topic of conversation, which seemed less of a topic of conversation with our teachers. I supposed I learned by example, by having good role models and some bad role models. Role models that I felt I very much I wanted to imitate, I would like to be like them. And other people I felt, my goodness me, I really would like to avoid being like that particular person.'

'And I am sure that's the same for a lot of medical students today, they are looking at their teachers and they . . .'

'. . . I'm sure, and I think some teachers underestimate their importance as a role model really.'

'So you went into general practice quite soon after qualifying, and you were in general practice in the 60s. In the 60s there would have been a lot of developments in general practice, do you want to tell me about that?'

'Yes, general practice, has always been, always seen itself as holistic subject, and in the 60s we were in many ways at that time not very satisfied with how we were developing as a dis-cipline. And we started thinking ourselves more as holistic doctors, making diagnosis in physical and emotional terms. We were very much influenced, at least in north London, by [Michael] Balint, who made us focus on the patient-doctor interactions. And looking at how we felt when we saw a patient. How did patients make us feel and how useful was that feeling that we got in reaching the diagnosis and helping us manage the patients. So we always had, developed a holistic approach.'

'So, in general practice at least, and in north London at least, you were quite ahead of the game in terms of focusing on the psychosocial aspects of the patient, its effects on you and those sort of things?'

'Yes. We set up a group for example where I practised, of young principles, people who just recently entered general practice and we met every month, to talk about difficult consultations and how we managed them and also we had some disease focused discussions as well, but most of the discussions were on the dynamics of the consultation.'

'So what are your thoughts about the differences between medical education now and 50 years ago?'

'Well we learned communication skills on the hoof, as I explained earlier on, now there's a much more professional approach to teaching communication skills. We're taught how to, medical students are taught how to, to talk to patients and the many different circumstances, from many different backgrounds. I think the whole approach to medical education is more patient-centred: 'What does the patient think? How does the patient react?' – than it was when I entered medical school. I also think that there is quite a big difference in the type of students who enter medical school, who apply to medical school.'

'...More women...'

'...More women, ethnically much more mixed. Unfortunately, and I think it is unfortunate, they still come from, I think, a similar social background, from the medical students who entered medical school 50 years ago, namely a professional background. Not always representing the background of the patients they are going to treat.'

'Thanks very much that's been very helpful. Thank you.'

Transcript of Peter's podcast

Go to www.oxfordtextbooks.co.uk/orc/washer/ to listen to the audio recording of this interview.

'Hello. My name is Peter Washer and I'm the editor of Clinical Communication Skills. I'm joined in this podcast by Mr Peter Kemble. Peter, tell me something about yourself.'

'My name is Peter Kemble, I'm 61 years old, and I'm severely disabled.'

'Okay, so I understand that you had a very nasty experience four years ago. Tell me briefly about that, because it's a very long story, but tell briefly me the upshot of it.'

'Okay, well I went to the hospital with an abscess on my behind. After going to the hospital several times, it turned to gangrene. I was then diagnosed as being diabetic, admitted, had seven major operations. Everything that could go wrong went wrong. I was in hospital for two months. I was released and was bed-bound for a year and during that time I couldn't get the information from the hospital of what had actually happened to me. The only way I could do this was go to a solicitor and get my notes.'

'Okay, so can I just sort of explore that? You were saying that after you'd been discharged from hospital, you were telling me earlier that you couldn't actually remember what had happened in hospital, it was bit of a blur, so you wanted to find out what exactly had happened. So you asked them to tell you and . . .'

'Yeah, I rang up the hospital and I asked for my notes, which they refused. The only way I could get that information was to get a solicitor and do it through the legal process.'

'Okay, so when you went to see the solicitor that was the goal, to get your notes?'

'Yeah, just to find out what had happened, yeah.'

'Right, and what happened when you . . . how long did it take to . . .'

'It took my solicitor six months to get my notes. Then we had to have them translated so that I could understand them, and then it was obvious that things had gone wrong. My solicitor advised me to sue them. I didn't want to sue them, I just wanted an explanation. I couldn't get an explanation from them, so I ended up suing them.'

'Okay. So if you had . . . right at the start, if they had given you your notes or sat down and explained exactly what had happened, do you think that you would have ended up suing them?'

'No, all I wanted to know was what had actually happened to me and why. That's all I wanted.'

'So what ultimately happened with the court case?'

'After them denying any wrong doing for four years, they settled five days before the court case.'

'So you did get money?'

'Yes I got £180,000.'

'Right, okay – that's quite a lot of money, isn't it?'

'But they still never apologised or said sorry.'

'So at the outset you weren't actually after money, you were after?'

'I just wanted an explanation . . .'

'. . . an explanation . . . and an apology?'

'Well obviously if they had made mistakes, if they could have explained that. I understand we all make mistakes. All they had to do was explain it, 'This person made a mistake', okay, fine, that's life. The thing wasn't about money; I just wanted to know what had happened to me. I was brought up with the belief that the National Health Service was a service; there to help me and to inform you and they didn't do that with me. They kept me in the dark.'

'And so you ended up in this situation of being involved in litigation which took many years?'

'Four years.'

'That was very expensive from their perspective.'

'Yeah, it was very expensive from everybody's perspective – and pointless. If they paid out money – I didn't go in it for money. If they paid their lawyers – they didn't need to have lawyers. All I needed was . . . The actual doctors I saw at the outpatients, they were

brilliant. They told me basically, 'We can't tell you anything, because the lawyers say we can't', but if was down to them they would.'

'If there'd been a proper explanation before you got to the solicitor, then the whole thing wouldn't have spun in that direction?'

'No of course not. When I first rung up the hospital and asked what had happened to me, if they'd just explained what had happened to me, that wouldn't have been that. You know, a year of lying in bed, trying to recover, and not knowing what had actually been done to me. I've got all these scars and wounds and I didn't know what they were for.'

'Thank you very much for that Peter, that was really, really helpful. Thank you.'

'Okay.'

Transcript of Roisin's podcast

Go to www.oxfordtextbooks.co.uk/orc/washer/ to listen to the audio recording of this interview.

'Hello my name is Peter Washer, and I'm the editor of Clinical Communication Skills and I am joined in this podcast by Roisin. Roisin thank you for talking to me, tell me a bit about yourself.'

'My name is Roisin, I am a pharmacist, I was age 41 when I was diagnosed with breast cancer about a year ago. My mother had died of breast cancer about four years previously and it was about three weeks before I was getting married that the diagnosis was made at London teaching hospital, as a result of me finding a lump and going to my GP, and having a referral to the teaching hospital.'

'So obviously a really terrible combination of circumstances. And as a result of getting diagnosed you had a lumpectomy. I am particularly interested in what the treatment options you were presented with after that. Can you tell me about that?'

'Initially I saw the consultant as a result of conversations with the breast-care nurse in relation to assisted fertility issues, because as I said I was just about to get married, I hadn't any children and we had been planning on starting a family, so I saw the consultant to put the issues of my treatment in the context of fertility, assisted fertility issues.'

' . . . and what were the options?'

'The options offered to me were, I had them presented to me in terms of the success rate: as a result of surgery; surgery plus radiotherapy; surgery plus radiotherapy and hormone treatment, because the cancer was an oestrogen-based tumour; or surgery radiotherapy and chemotherapy.'

'So increasing in the success rates, the latter ones being the highest?'

'Yes, I mean the success rate, if I had selected the option of chemotherapy combined with radiotherapy and surgery was 1% greater than if I had gone for the hormone-based treatment combined with radiotherapy and surgery. But then it was put in the context of far fewer extreme side-effects.'

'Sure, so did you come away from that consultation with the sense that the doctor and the breast care team were favouring a particular option?'

'Yes I did. I felt they were favouring the hormone-based treatment combined with radiotherapy and surgery because it had a higher success rate. I think at the time they said it had 95% , but it had far fewer side-effects than if I had opted for the chemotherapy which had a slightly, I think a 1%, higher success rate but significantly more side effects, so I came away feeling that was the option that was being sort of highly recommended, it was still put it in the context of it being my choice.'

'Right, but that was the one you chose?'

'Yes it was the one I chose.'

'So kind of begs the question, why did you trust them with taking the option that they were favouring. What was it about them?'

'From the start, from my experience within healthcare and the NHS, I was aware that the outcomes for patients being treated at teaching hospitals are better than non-teaching hospitals. This was a leading London teaching hospital. The consultant himself was very knowledgeable, didn't patronise me, pitched the information at a level that I felt was appropriate, and there was a very, very integrated approach of the breast-care nurses, and from the start there was a dedicated breast-care unit there. I felt that the consultants and all the associated staff worked very well together as a team and I felt that my particular case, the consultant had mentioned that he'd looked at the information in my patient records and had plotted sort of statistics and this was the option they were recommending, and I felt that my specific circumstances had been put in context of wider population studies.'

'So, it is a whole series of things about the institution and the team, particular individuals within that and you felt you were being treated as an individual but within the whole thing, all these things were really reassuring enough for you to follow their advice?'

'Yes.'

'One last thing I wanted to ask you about: because you are a pharmacist, did you feel that the information was pitched at the right level for you, because you obviously are not a lay member of the public?'

'I do. I think because the reason that I initially saw the consultant for the first time, the oncology consultant, is because the issues around assisted fertility had come up and there was uncertainty as to whether the high dose of oestrogen that would be used as part of the ovarian stimulation would have an impact on the tumour, particularly because there was going to be a gap for the fertility treatment between the surgery and the start of either radiotherapy or the treatment. So I felt the questions that I was asking pitched the conversation at a level that the consultant then responded I felt appropriately with information.'

'So, I mean, he was responding to the questions you were asking and that was why the level was right because you kind of gave them permission to pitch it at that level right from the start.'

'Yes because, I think, the meeting had been set up by the breast-care nurse specifically to answer these queries and I felt that any of the questions that I came up with he was able to provide what I felt were informed answers and confident responses.'

'OK, that's great, Thank you very much for that.'

'It's a pleasure.'

Transcript of Sam's podcast

Go to www.oxfordtextbooks.co.uk/orc/washer/ to listen to the audio recording of this interview.

'Hello, I'm Peter Washer and I am the editor of Clinical Communication Skills, and I am joined today by Dr Caroline Fertleman, who is a consultant paediatrician at the Whittington Hospital in north London, and by Sam, who is a patient, and Debbie, his mum. Welcome. Sam, tell me a little bit about yourself.'

'Well, I've got thallassemia because I haven't many blood cells in my body.'

'And how old are you?'

'Eight going on nine.'

'And you've had this for a long time?'

'Yes, about eight years.'

'So you've got a lot of experience of being in and out of hospitals and doctors, too much experience probably. So tell me what's been your experience of doctors talking to you?'

'The doctors have been really nice by asking me if I am okay.'

'So tell me more about when they're nice, what do they do?'

'They explain things to me.'

'Is there anything else?'

'No.'

'OK, you talked to me a bit before Sam about once, when you went to your GP when you had sore ears. Can you tell me about what happened there and about how the doctor communicated, talked to you?'

'She explained to my mum and asked me if it hurt in some places in my body and she checked me.'

'And when the doctor was talking to you was he looking at you, at your mum or both, how did it work?'

'She was looking at mainly at my mum and looked at me sometimes.'

'And who did he talked to?'

'Mostly my mum.'

'And was that ok or did you wish he would have talked to you more?'

'It was fine.'

'Mum, can I ask you, what have been your experiences? Obviously you've been around with Sam a lot around hospitals and doctors, tell me more how it has been for you.'

'Because of Sam's condition every doctor I have been to has been absolutely fine. They've explained to us about the condition, they've explained to us about the medication, they've explained to us about the problems, they've explained to us the good things and the bad things and the type of things to look out for. So my experience have been absolutely excellent at the hospital and the doctors.

'Obviously being a parent of a sick child is very, very stressful, very anxiety provoking, so tell me, you were saying earlier about how it was when you first found out that Sam had thalassemia, so tell me more about that.'

'The doctor that I saw, I sort of started crying when I found out about the condition, sort of snapped me out of it and told me that I mustn't cry and I must be strong for my child. And to be honest with you it was the best thing that could have happened. I did snap out of it, and did pull myself together and I had to accept, I had to learn to accept still to be honest with you, you have to get on with it, to be honest with you, the doctor put me straight and said no crying you have to look after your child.'

'So okay, I don't want to put words in your mouth, but it sounds like the doctor was kind of strong for you?'

'The doctor was harsh, but for me personally it was the best thing I needed, for some people it could have broken them, for me it was the best thing I needed. Otherwise I would have carried on crying to this day. But it was the best thing I needed. And then you start to listen to what the doctors have to say, you understand and you have to start the medication to be honest with you.'

'And the explanations that you've had, have they been right amount and right level and so on?'

'Yes, and if I needed to know more and ask questions I get told the answer straight away. As far as I know they don't leave anything out, for all the questions that I have asked I've had an answer to.'

'And you were saying earlier that when they explain things to you it's with Sam there. Is not like they ask to speak to you separately?'

'No, never.'

'And that is good as far as you are concerned?'

'I think so. I think he should be aware, yes. If you hide then they ask questions I think he would be more shocked, I think he should be aware, yes.'

'Have you got any questions Caroline?'

'Have the doctors always explained things or do you explain things to Sam, if they are talking to you rather than him?'

'The doctors talk to both of us, I notice they look at Sam and they look at me, but they tend to explain more to me. If he doesn't understand, on the way home he asks questions and I explain them it to him after-wards. So he might not say doctor I did not understand, he waits until we get home and then he would say to me, 'I didn't understand Mum can you tell me?' But the doctors try to explain, we are always together, and they always try to explain to both of us.'

'And have you found it's changed over the time he has got older because he started having this condition when he was a baby and he now nearly nine. Have you seen a change in how they . . . ?'

'I have, I have because at the beginning the doctor always spoke to me, whereas now they look at my son, they ask him and they check him and they ask him. Say like if he needs an MRI, they ask him they explain him what it is, and they look at him and talk to him. They have changed, the doctors, because now is getting older they talk to him more. I think they do it is just he does not understand so much all the medical terms which is we then explain to him.'

'So, have you got any sort of take home messages for medical students, future doctors in terms of the way parents and children should be . . . ?'

'Talk to the child, ask them if they understand and they explain in simple terms. You know like when he was told he needed an MRI, the doctor, he just said, "What's an MRI?" which is fair enough because at 8 years old he wouldn't know. And the doctor explained better that I would have explained, how simple it is. Just talk to the child and ask them if they understand, that's important.'

'And is there anything you would like to say to future doctors Sam?'

'No.'

'No you haven't. Okay thank you both very much.'

'Thank you.'

'Thank you.'

Transcript of Valerie's podcast

Go to www.oxfordtextbooks.co.uk/orc/washer/ to listen to the audio recording of this interview.

'Hello my name is Peter Washer, I'm the editor of Clinical Communication Skills and in this podcast I am joined by Valerie. Valerie tell me about yourself.'

'I am 48 years old, I am a mother of 12 year old son and I discovered I was HIV positive in 1985.'

'OK, so 1985 is quite early on in the AIDS epidemic, what were the circumstances of you getting that test?'

'My grandmother was having an operation for stomach cancer, and the hospital was asking relatives for blood for their blood bank of the hospital.'

'So you were tested in order to give for the blood transfusion for your grandmother. Most people who go along for an HIV test kind of expect that they might be positive, that's why they go and get tested. Was that the case with you? Did you have any suspicions?'

'I had unprotected sex and I 'played' a little bit with syringes, but I was hoping not . . .'

'Sure, sure, you said you had unprotected sex . . .'

'I had opportunity to catch it.'

'Sure. Now what was the situation with the counselling for the test?'

'When the result arrived eight weeks after, the doctor told me straightaway, a doctor I had never saw before, told me straightaway 'You've got AIDS'. At that time there was no difference between HIV and AIDS, and they left the room to leave me to cope with this news. Of course I was feeling almost dead. I was giving myself three months to live and three months after instead there I was self destructive, using more drugs and using more drink.'

'What you are saying is that as a result of test being handled really badly by the doctor's communication skills you ended up getting even more self destructive in the immediate period afterwards?'

'Yes, nobody was asking me how I was feeling, it was only come to the hospital once a month to have a blood test and we'll tell you the answer next month when you come in, but I don't know what the answer was I don't know what they were looking for.'

'That was a very long time ago, 23 years ago, and you are still well, and you've since moved to London, and you are now with a London teaching hospital as your HIV treatment centre. So in contrast to that experience, which was really terrible, you seem to have a good relationship now with your HIV treatment centre. Tell me what's good about them?'

'The centre where I go covers all aspects. As an HIV person you have to look at the globality of the person, and if I have not only physical problem but also depression problems, housing problems, my son problems, I always, have someone to give a shoulder to cry or ears to listen.'

'OK, a big part of what is good about the relationship you've got with the HIV centre now, is just that you've been with them for quite a few years so it is a long relationship and they are available for you, does that sound . . . ?'

'Yes, they try to be available if I need without appointment and if I need to see a counsellor because of some reasons, I'm sure I find a counsellor, the counsellor will find, even between appointments, time for me. And I don't feel judged if I go for a . . . if I make a mistake in my life, I don't feel judged, I don't feel to hide, I don't need to hide to them my mistakes in life.'

'So you feel that them being non-judgmental is really important and that is one of the things that make your relationship with them now good. OK, is there anything else you would like to say to medical students who are listening to this?'

'I like my HIV [treatment centre] because the doctors are more direct, more straight, they don't fiddle around with questions. If they want to know if I use the syringes they ask me 'Did you use syringes?' they didn't ask 'How did you get it?' and also they give me, they teach me what is about the HIV, what we have a blood test for, what . . . and everything.'

'So they explain to you?'

'Exactly.'

'That is very important as well.'

'They explain to me my liver, my cells, my CDAs (CD4) all the stuff. Before now, I was giving blood and I didn't know what they were looking for.'

'And because you had these explanations you understand what is going on and that presumably makes you feel more in control of . . . ?'

'Yes, it makes me feel more in control, and don't make me lie to the doctors. There is no reason, because they, I grow up with the doctors and it's better for me and in fact after so many years I don't take any combination [therapy], I took some AZT during my pregnancy and my son also is [HIV] negative and that's it.'

'OK thank you, that's really, really helpful.'

Links to websites

Web addresses

General

The Calgary Cambridge Model
This is the website relating to Kurtz (in Calgary) and
Silverman (in Cambridge) and their influential clinical communication model
http://www.skillscascade.com/index.html

UK Postgraduate Medical Education and Training Board
PMETB is the regulatory body responsible for postgraduate medical education and training in the UK,
responsible for establishing national standards and
requirements for postgraduate medical education
and training; making sure these standards and
requirements are met and developing and promoting
postgraduate medical education.
http://www.pmetb.org.uk/index.php?id=10

Communicating With Your Doctor: The PACE System
This interesting US site is aimed at patients, and gives
them advice on how to best communicate with their
doctors
http://patcom.jcomm.ohio-state.edu/preface.htm

Chapter 6 Talking with disabled people

British Sign Language
This site uses moving pictures to give some basic words
in British Sign Language
http://www.britishsignlanguage.com/

Hearing Concern Link
UK charity providing support for deaf and hearing
impaired people. Their website is mostly aimed at
people affected by hearing impairment.
http://www.hearingconcernlink.org/

Mencap
Mencap is a UK learning disability charity working with
people with a learning disability and their families
and carers. Their website includes links to a range of
resources for professional and lay audiences.
http://www.mencap.org.uk/

Easyinfo
This is a site for those working with people with
learning difficulties and for people with learning
difficulties themselves and aims to make information
easier for people with learning difficulties.
www.easyinfo.org.uk

Royal National Institute of Blind People (RNIB)
UK based charity offering advice and support to people
with sight loss. Their website includes a range of
links to related resources
http://www.rnib.org.uk/
The RNIB site includes a particularly useful section on
how to guide people with sight problems
http://www.rnib.org.uk/xpedio/groups/public/
documents/publicwebsite/public_howtoguide.hcsp

Royal National Institute for Deaf People (RNID)
Includes factsheets for patients, as well as information
resources for health professionals
http://www.rnid.org.uk/

Sense

Sense is a UK charity that supports and campaigns for children and adults who are deafblind. Their website has a range of resources, including useful information for health professionals on how to help and advise people who are deafblind.

http://www.sense.org.uk/

More information about deafblind manual alphabet can be found at http://www.sense.org.uk/aboutdeaf-blindness/communication/deafblind_manual.htm

There is also a video clip at this address demonstrating how to use deafblind manual alphabet.

Speakability

Speakability is a UK charity that supports and empowers people with Aphasia. Their website has a range of useful resources, mostly aimed at people with aphasia rather than health professionals.

http://www.speakability.org.uk/

The British Stammering Organisation

http://www.stammering.org/

This website includes a useful guide to talking with people who stammer

http://www.stammering.org/conversation.html

The UK Equality and Human Rights Commission

UK Government's website on Disability, with loads of information on the law related to disability etc

http://www.equalityhumanrights.com/en/yourrights/equalityanddiscrimination/disability/

Valuing People

Valuing People is the UK government's plan for making the lives of people with learning disabilities, their families and carers better. The website has a resources section where there are hundreds of papers relevant to people with learning disabilities and links to other peoples' websites, organised by subject area.

http://valuingpeople.gov.uk/index.jsp

Clinical Communication with People with Learning Disabilities

This site is hosted by St Georges Hospital Medical School and gives practical advice on how to communicate with people with a learning disability.

http://www.intellectualdisability.info/how_to/clin_comms.htm

Disability Rights Education and Defense Fund

US civil rights law and policy centre directed by individuals with disabilities and parents who have children with disabilities

http://www.dredf.org/index.shtml

Leonard Cheshire Disability

UK based disability charity, part of a Global Alliance of non-governmental organisations in 52 countries, with regional offices based in Asia, Africa, Latin America and Caribbean

http://www.lcdisability.org/

Enable

The United Nations Secretariat for the Convention on the Rights of Persons with Disabilities

http://www.un.org/disabilities/index.asp

Chapter 7 Talking with people from other cultures

NHS Equality and Diversity

The UK NHS Equality and Diversity website has information and links to issues related to NHS staff, such as about disciplinary procedures and whistle blowing.

http://www.nhsemployers.org/excellence/equality-diversity.cfm

Chapter 9 Talking with children and young people

Action for Sick Children

UK's largest charity dedicated to caring for sick children, their website includes a section on information for health professionals

http://www.actionforsickchildren.org/

Information Sharing

UK Department for Education and Skills Practitioners' Guide describing UK 'Every Child Matters' policy

http://www.everychildmatters.gov.uk/deliveringservices/informationsharing/

What to do if you're worried a child is being abused

UK government policy on dealing with child abuse from the Department of Education and Skills.

http://www.everychildmatters.gov.uk/resources-and-practice/IG00182/

Working Together to Safeguard Children

This is the UK government's policy that sets out how individuals and organisations should work together to safeguard and promote the welfare of children.

http://www.everychildmatters.gov.uk/resources-and-practice/IG00060/

National Society for the Prevention of Cruelty to Children (NSPCC)
UK Child Protection charity.
http://www.nspcc.org.uk/

Royal College of Paediatrics and Child Health
RCPCH guidance on Safeguarding Children and Young People: Roles and competences for health care staff.
http://www.rcpch.ac.uk/Health-Services/
Child-Protection/Child-Protection-Publications

The Society for Adolescent Medicine
SAM is a US multi-disciplinary organization of health professionals who are committed to advancing the health and well-being of adolescents. Their website has a range of health related resources for health professionals, for teenagers and their parents.
http://www.adolescenthealth.org/

European Training in Effective Adolescent Care and Health (EuTEACH) Programme
This site was developed for use by health care professionals involved in either the teaching of adolescent health or clinical care of adolescents and young adults.
http://www.euteach.com/

Chapter 10 Talking with people with mental health problems

Alcohol Concern
UK National Agency on alcohol misuse, includes a range of alcohol related resources and factsheets
www.alcoholconcern.org.uk

Drink Aware
An independent UK charity that campaigns to change people's drinking habits for the better. Website includes a range of alcohol-related fact sheets
www.drinkaware.co.uk

Stand to Reason
Stand to Reason is a UK based lobbying group fighting discrimination and stigma, challenging stereotypes and changing attitudes relating to mental health. Their website has more information about their campaigns.
http://standtoreason.org.uk/home

Sane
Sane is a UK charity that aims to raise awareness and respect for people with mental illness and their families, undertake research into the causes of serious mental illness and provide help and information to those experiencing mental health problems, their families and carers. Their website has a range of factsheets, research reports and other resources aimed at lay people and health professionals.
http://www.sane.org.uk/

Hearing Voices Network
A UK organisation started by patients and carers, which provides opportunities for people experiencing psychotic symptoms to talk about them
http://www.hearing-voices.org/

Talk to Frank
UK government advice and information service about all drugs
www.talktofrank.com
And related site specifically about cannabis
www.knowcannabis.org.uk

Chapter 13 Talking about mistakes and dealing with complaints

The NHS Litigation Authority
The NHSLA is a Special Health Authority (part of the British National Health Service), responsible for handling negligence claims made against NHS bodies in England. Their web site has an section on advice for clinicians, as well as information for patients
http://www.nhsla.com/

The National Patient Safety Agency
The NPSA is an 'arms length' agency of the UK Department of Health, with a remit to improve patient safety by reporting and enabling the NHS to learn from safety incidents. Their website includes links to a range of reports on medication and surgical safety etc
http://www.npsa.nhs.uk/

Being Open when Patients are Harmed
UK National Patient Safety Organisation's policy document relating to apologising to patients harmed in adverse events
http://www.npsa.nhs.uk/nrls/alerts-and-directives/notices/disclosure/

Chapter 14 Shared decision making and communicating risk

UK Cancer screening programmes
This site has information on UK screening programmes for breast, bowel and cervical cancer, as well as a link to an informed choice management tool on prostate cancer
http://www.cancerscreening.nhs.uk/index.html

Risk Charts for Cancer Risk

See: Woloshin S, Schwartz LM, Welch HG Risk Charts: Putting Cancer in Context (2002) Journal of the National Cancer Institute 94 (11) p799 – 804 Available online at http://jncicancerspectrum.oupjournals.org/cgi/content/full/jnci;94/11/799 This paper contains simple charts with age, sex and smoking-specific data about the chance of dying from various common causes in the next ten years.

Detailed epidemiological data on time-frame and life-time risks

From UK NHS National Library for Health http://www.library.nhs.uk/

This site is aimed at Health Professionals, although includes different levels of information for patients, including a comprehensive library of patient information leaflets at http://cks.library.nhs.uk/patient_information

Dr Chris Cates Evidence-Based Medicine Site

This is a website which can help interpret results from systematic reviews and clinical trials. It includes free downloadable software which can convert Odds Ratios into Numbers Needed to Treat, and produces graphical displays demonstrating the impact of treatment if it were given to 100 people with the relevant condition.

www.nntonline.net

The Cochrane Library of Patient Decision Aids

As described in the book, this site based at the Ottowa Health Research Institute contains a comprehensive library range of patient decision aids, and uses international standards to rate their quality.

www.ohri.ca/decisionaid

Your Disease Risk

Hosted at the Washington University Medical School, this website has personalized risk information (for patients) on developing cancer, stroke, diabetes, osteoporosis and heart disease and personalized tips for helping to prevent them.

http://www.yourdiseaserisk.wustl.edu/

Cancer Risk Assessment Tool

Based at the Memorial Sloan Kettering Cancer Centre this website is aimed at health professionals and patients and gives tailored risk estimates for a variety of different cancers.

http://www.mskcc.org/mskcc/html/5794.cfm

Breast Cancer Risk Assessment Tool

The US National Cancer Institute website, aimed at health professionals http://www.cancer.gov/bcrisk-tool/

References

Visit the online resource centre for *Clinical Communication Skills* at: www.oxfordtextbooks.co.uk/orc/washer where you will find active web links to the *majority* of the sources listed below. The editor selected these supporting references, having completed an extensive literature review (spanning over 1000 papers) to underpin the writing of this book.

In most cases, you will be able to view the abstract readily, and depending on what level of access you or your institution has to individual online journal content, you may be able to click through directly to the full article. By presenting links in this way, we hope to provide you with a helpful gateway to a collection of core communication skills literature, in order to guide your onward reading and provide a starting point for assignments and literature searches.

Abdel-Tawab, N. and Roter, D. (2002). The relevance of client-centered communication to family planning settings in developing countries: Lessons from the Egyptian experience. *Social Science and Medicine*, **54**(9), 1357–1368.

Aggleton, P., Oliver, C., and Rivers, K. (1998). *Reducing the Rate of Teenage Conceptions. The Implications of Research into Young People, Sex, Sexuality and Relationships.* London: The Health Education Authority.

Akabayashi, A., Kai, I., Takemura, H., and Okazaki, H. (1999). Truth telling in the case of a pessimistic diagnosis in Japan. *The Lancet*, **354**(9186), 1263.

Album, D. and Westin, S. (2008). Do diseases have a prestige hierarchy? A survey among physicians and medical students. *Social Science and Medicine*, **66**, 182–188.

Alcohol Concern (2001). *Screening Tools for Healthcare Settings.* Primary Care Alcohol Information Service London: Alcohol Concern.

Ali, N., Atkin, K., and Neal, R. (2006). The role of culture in the general practice consultation process. *Ethnicity and Health*, **11**(4), 389–408.

Ambady, N., Laplante, D., Nguyen, T., Rosenthal, R., Chaumeton, N., and Levinson, W. (2002). Surgeons' tone of voice: A clue to malpractice history. *Surgery*, **132**(1), 5–9.

Aquilina, C. and Warner, J. (2004). *A Guide to Psychiatric Examination.* Knutsford, UK: Pastest.

Arborelius, E. and Bremberg, S. (1992). What can doctors do to achieve a successful consultation? Videotaped interviews analysed by the 'consultation map' method. *Family Practice*, **9**(1), 61–67.

Aspegren, K. and Lonberg-Masden, P. (2005). Which basic communication skills in medicine are learnt spontaneously and which need to be taught and trained? *Medical Teacher*, **27**(6), 539–543.

Association of American Medical Colleges (1999). *Contemporary Issues in Medicine: Communication in Medicine.* Washington DC: AAMC.

Baile, W.F., Kudelka, A.P., Beale, E.A., Glober, G.A., Myers, E.G., Greisinger, A.J., Bast, R.C., Jr., Goldstein, M.G., Novack, D., and Lenzi, R. (1999). Communication skills training in oncology. Description and preliminary outcomes of workshops on breaking bad news and managing patient reactions to illness. *Cancer*, **86**(5), 887–897.

Baile, W., Buckman, R., Lenzi, R., Glober, G., Beale, E., and Kudelka, A. (2000). SPIKES – A six-step protocol for delivering bad news: Application to the patient with cancer. *The Oncologist*, **5**(4), 302–311.

Balint, M. (1964). *The Doctor, his Patient and the Illness*. London: Pitman Medical.

Barnes, J. (2003). Quality, efficacy and safety of complementary medicines: Fashions, facts and the future. Part II: Efficacy and safety. *British Journal of Clinical Pharmacology*, **55**, 331–340.

Barnett, M. (2002). Effect of breaking bad news on patients' perceptions of doctors. *Journal of the Royal Society of Medicine*, **95**(7), 343–347.

Barnett, P.B. (2001). Rapport and the hospitalist. *The American Journal of Medicine*, **111**(9B), 31S–35S.

Barry, C.A., Bradley, C.P., Britten, N., Stevenson, F.A., and Barber, N. (2000). Patients' unvoiced agendas in general practice consultations: Qualitative study. *British Medical Journal*, **320**(7244), 1246–1250.

Barsky, A.J. (1988). *Worried Sick: Our Troubled Quest for Wellness*. Boston and Toronto: Little, Brown and Company.

Bass, L.W. and Cohen, R.L. (1982). Ostensible versus actual reasons for seeking pediatric attention: Another look at the parental ticket of admission. *Pediatrics*, **70**(6), 870–874.

Beaver, K., Luker, K.A., Owens, R.G., Leinster, S.J., Degner, L.F., and Sloan, J.A. (1996). Treatment decision making in women newly diagnosed with breast cancer. *Cancer Nursing*, **19**(1), 8–19.

Bell, R.A., Kravitz, R.L., Thom, D., Krupat, E., and Azari, R. (2002). Unmet expectations for care and the patient–physician relationship. *Journal of General Internal Medicine*, **17**(11), 817–824.

Bellaby, P. (2003). Communication and miscommunication of risk: Understanding UK parents' attitudes to combined MMR vaccination. *British Medical Journal*, **327**(7417), 725–728.

Benson, J. and Britten, N. (1996). Respecting the autonomy of cancer patients when talking with their families: Qualitative analysis of semi-structured interviews with patients. *British Medical Journal*, **313**(7059), 729–731.

Bligh, J. (1999). Persistent attenders and heartsink. *Medical Education*, **33**(6), 398.

BMA Board of Medical Education (2004). *Communication Skills Education for Doctors: An Update*. London: British Medical Association.

Bonvicini, K. and Perlin, M. (2003). The same but different: Clinician–patient communication with gay and lesbian patients. *Patient Education and Counselling*, **51**, 115–122.

Bridson, J., Hammond, C., Leach, A., and Chester, M. (2003). Making consent patient centred. *British Medical Journal*, **327**(7424), 1159–1161.

Bristol Royal Infirmary Inquiry (2001). The Bristol Royal Infirmary Inquiry. London: HMSO.

British Medical Association (2004a). *Medical Certificates and Reports*. London: British Medical Association.

British Medical Association (2004b). *Safe Handover, Safe Patients. Guidance on Clinical Handover for Cinicians and Managers*. London: British Medical Association.

Brown, J. (2008). How clinical communication has become a core part of medical education in the UK. *Medical Education*, **42**, 271–278.

Burack, J.H., Irby, D.M., Carline, J.D., Root, R.K., and Larson, E.B. (1999). Teaching compassion and respect: Attending physicians' responses to problematic behaviors. *Journal of General Internal Medicine*, **14**(1), 49–55.

Burkitt Wright, E., Holcombe, C., and Salmon, P. (2004). Doctors' communication of trust, care, and respect in breast cancer: Qualitative study. *British Medical Journal*, **328**(7444), 864–868.

Butow, P.N., Dunn, S.M., Tattersall, M.H.N., and Jones, Q.J. (1994). Patient participation in the cancer consultation; Evaluation of a question prompt sheet. *Annals of Oncology*, **5**(3), 199–204.

Butow, P.N., Brown, R.F., Cogar, S., Tattersall, M.H., and Dunn, S.M. (2002). Oncologists' reactions to cancer patients' verbal cues. *Psychooncology*, **11**(1), 47–58.

Byron, M., Howell, C., Bradley, P., Bheenuck, S., Wickham, C., and Curran, T. (2006). *Different Differences: Disability Equality Teaching in Healthcare Education*. Bristol: University of Bristol, University of the West of England, and Peninsula Medical School.

Calman, K. and Royston, G. (1997). Risk language and dialects. *British Medical Journal*, **315**(7113), 939–942.

Car, J. and Sheikh, A. (2003). Telephone consultations. *British Medical Journal*, **326**(7396), 966–969.

Carr, S. (2006). The Foundation Programme assessment tools: An opportunity to enhance feedback to trainees? *Postgraduate Medical Journal*, **82**(576), 579.

Cave, J. and Dacre, J. (2008). Dealing with complaints. *British Medical Journal*, **336**, 326–336.

Charles, C., Gafni, A., and Whelan, T. (1997). Shared decision-making in the medical encounter: What does it mean? (or it takes at least two to tango). *Social Science and Medicine*, **44**(5), 681–692.

Charles, C., Gafni, A., and Whelan, T. (1999). Decision-making in the physician–patient encounter: Revisiting the shared treatment decision-making model. *Social Science and Medicine*, **49**(5), 651–661.

Christakis, N. and Lamont, E. (2000). Extent and determinants of error in doctors' prognoses in terminally ill patients: Prospective cohort study. *British Medical Journal*, **320**(7233), 469–473.

Christie, D. and Viner, R. (2005). Adolescent development. *British Medical Journal*, **330**(7486), 301–304.

Cockayne, N., Duguid, M., and Shenfield, G. (2004). Health professionals rarely record history of complementary and alternative medicines. *British Journal of Clinical Pharmacology*, **59**(2), 254–258.

Constable, S., Ham, A., and Pirmohamed, M. (2006). Herbal medicines and acute medical emergency admissions to hospital. *British Journal of Clinical Pharmacology*, **63**(2), 247–248.

Coulehan, J.L., Platt, F.W., Egener, B., Frankel, R., Lin, C.T., Lown, B., and Salazar, W.H. (2001). 'Let me see if I have this right . . .': Words that help build empathy. *Annals of Internal Medicine*, **135**(3), 221–227.

Coulter, A. (1999). Paternalism or partnership? Patients have grown up – and there's no going back. *British Medical Journal*, **319**(7212), 719–720.

Coulter, A., Entwistle, V., & Gilbert, D. (1999). Sharing decisions with patients: Is the information good enough? *British Medical Journal*, **318**(7179), 318–322.

Cox, L. and Roper, T. (2005). *Clinical Skills*. Oxford: Oxford University Press.

Cunningham, V., Lefkoe, M., and Sechrest, L. (2006). Eliminating fears: An intervention that permanently eliminates the fear of public speaking. *Clinical Psychology and Psychotherapy*, **13**(3), 183–193.

Dalton, P. (1994). *Counselling People with Communication Problems*. London: Sage Publications.

Davies, T. (1997). ABC of mental health: Mental health assessment. *British Medical Journal*, **314**(7093), 1536–1539.

De Smet, P. (2006). Clinical risk management of herb–drug interactions. *British Journal of Clinical Pharmacology*, **63**(3), 258–267.

Department of Health (2002a). *Building a Safer NHS for Patients: Implementing an Organisation with a Memory*. London: HMSO.

Department of Health (2002b). *Learning from Bristol: the Department of Health's Response to the Report of the Public Inquiry into Children's Heart Surgery at the Bristol Royal Infirmary 1984–1995*. London: HMSO.

Department of Health (2004). *Committee of Inquiry – Independent Investigation into How the NHS Handled Allegations about the Conduct of Clifford Ayling*. London: HMSO.

Department of Health (2005a). *The Kerr / Haslam Inquiry: Full Report*. London: HMSO.

Department of Health (2005b). *The Shipman Inquiry: Independent Public Inquiry into the Issues Arising from the Case of Harold Frederick Shipman*. London: HMSO.

Department of Health Expert Group (2000). *An Organisation with a Memory*. London: HMSO.

Department of Health NSW (2007). *Open Disclosure Guidelines*. North Sydney, NSW: Department of Health, NSW.

Diamond, J. (2001). *Snake Oil and Other Preoccupations*. London: Vintage.

Dosanjh, S., Barnes, J., and Bhandari, M. (2001). Barriers to breaking bad news among medical and surgical residents. *Medical Education*, **35**(3), 197–205.

Edwards, A. and Elwyn, G.J. (2001). Risks – Listen and don't mislead. *British Journal of General Practice*, **51**(465), 259–260.

Edwards, A., Matthews, E., Pill, R., and Bloor, M. (1998). Communication about risk: The responses of primary care professionals to standardizing the 'language of risk' and communication tools. *Family Practice*, **15**(4), 301–307.

Edwards, A., Elwyn, G., Covey, J., Matthews, E., and Pill, R. (2001). Presenting risk information – A review of the effects of 'framing' and other manipulations on patient outcomes. *Journal of Health Communication*, **6**(1), 61–82.

Edwards, A., Elwyn, G., and Mulley, A. (2002). Explaining risks: Turning numerical data into meaningful pictures. *British Medical Journal*, **324**(7341), 827–830.

Eggly, S., Penner, L., Albrecht, T., Cline, R., Foster, T., Naughton, M., Peterson, A., and Ruckdeschel, J. (2006). Discussing bad news in the outpatient oncology clinic: Rethinking current communication guidelines. *Journal of Clinical Oncology*, **24**(4), 716–719.

Ehrich, K. (2006). Telling cultures: 'Cultural' issues for staff reporting concerns about colleagues in the UK National Health Service. *Sociology of Health and Illness*, **28**(7), 903–926.

Elliot, D. and Hickam, D. (1997). How do faculty evaluate students' case presentations? *Teaching and Learning in Medicine*, **9**(4), 261–263.

Elwyn, G., Edwards, A., Gwyn, R., and Grol, R. (1999a). Towards a feasible model for shared decision making: Focus group study with general practice registrars. *British Medical Journal*, **319**(7212), 753–756.

Elwyn, G., Edwards, A., and Kinnersley, P. (1999b). Shared decision-making in primary care: The neglected second half of the consultation. *British Journal of General Practice*, **49**(443), 477–482.

Ende, J. (1983). Feedback in clinical medical education. *Journal of the American Medical Association*, **250**(6), 777–781.

Epstein, R.M., Morse, D.S., Frankel, R.M., Frarey, L., Anderson, K., and Beckman, H.B. (1998). Awkward moments in patient–physician communication about HIV risk. *Annals of Internal Medicine*, **128**(6), 435–442.

Epstein, R.M., Quill, T.E., and McWhinney, I.R. (1999). Somatization reconsidered: Incorporating the patient's experience of illness. *Archives of Internal Medicine*, **159**(3), 215–222.

Fallowfield, L. and Jenkins, V. (2004). Communicating sad, bad, and difficult news in medicine. *The Lancet*, **363**(9405), 312–319.

Fayers, T., Crowley, T., Jenkins, J., and Cahill, D. (2003). Medical student awareness of sexual health is poor. *International Journal of STD and AIDS*, **14**(6), 386–389.

Ferguson, W.J. and Candib, L.M. (2002). Culture, language, and the doctor-patient relationship. *Family Medicine*, **34**(5), 353–361.

Finlay, W., Antaki, C., and Walton, C. (2008). Saying no to the staff: An analysis of refusals in a home for people with severe communication difficulties. *Sociology of Health and Illness*, **30**(1), 55–75.

Fischer, M., Mazor, K., Baril, J., Alper, E., DeMarco, D., and Pugnaire, M. (2006). Learning from mistakes. *Journal of General Internal Medicine*, **21**, 419–423.

Fox, R. (1957). Training for uncertainty. In: R. Merton, G. Reader, and P. Kendall (Eds), *The Student Physician: Introductory Studies in the Sociology of Medical Education*. Cambridge, Massachusetts: Harvard University Press.

Frank, J., Jabbour, M., Tugwell, P., Boyd, D., Frechette, D., Labrosse, J., MacFayden, J., Marks, M., Neufield, V., Polson, A., Shea, B., Turnbull, J., and von Rosendaal, G. (1996). *Skills for the New Millennium: Report of the Societal Needs Working Group*. Ottawa: Royal College of Physicians and Surgeons of Canada.

Friedrichsen, M., Strang, P., and Carlsson, M. (2000). Breaking bad news in the transition from curative to palliative cancer care – Patient's view of the doctor giving the information. *Support Care Cancer*, **8**(6), 472–478.

Fugh-Berman, A. and Ernst, E. (2001). Herb–drug interactions: Review and assessment of report reliability. *British Journal of Clinical Pharmacology*, **52**, 587–595.

Gafaranga, J. and Britten, N. (2003). 'Fire away': The opening sequence in general practice consultations. *Family Practice*, **20**(3), 242–247.

Gattellari, M., Butow, P.N., and Tattersall, M.H. (2001). Sharing decisions in cancer care. *Social Science and Medicine*, **52**(12), 1865–1878.

General Medical Council (1993). *Tomorrow's Doctors*. London: GMC.

Gigerenzer, G. (2002). *Reckoning with Risk: Learning to Live with Uncertainty*. London: Allen Lane, The Penguin Press.

Gigerenzer, G. and Edwards, A. (2003). Simple tools for understanding risks: From innumeracy to insight. *British Medical Journal*, **327**(7417), 741–744.

Gill, D. and Sharpe, M. (1999). Frequent consulters in general practice: A systematic review of studies of prevalence, associations and outcome. *Journal of Psychosomatic Research*, **47**(2), 115–130.

Glendinning, E.H. and Holmstrom, B.A.S. (2005). *English in Medicine*, 3rd edn. Cambridge: Cambridge University Press.

Godolphin, W., Towle, A., and McKendry, R. (2001). Evaluation of the quality of patient information to support informed shared decision making. *Health Expectations*, **4**(4), 235–242.

Gott, M., Hinchliff, S., and Galena, E. (2004). General practitioner attitudes to discussing sexual health issues with older people. *Social Science and Medicine*, **58**(11), 2093–2103.

Greenberg, C., Regenbogen, S., Studdert, D., Lipsitz, S., Rogers, S., Zinner, M., and Gawande, A. (2007). Patterns of communication breakdowns resulting in injury to surgical patients. *Journal of the American College of Surgeons*, **204**(4), 533–540.

Greenhalgh, T., Voisey, C., and Robb, N. (2007). Interpreted consultations as 'business as usual'? An analysis of organisational routines in general practices. *Sociology of Health and Illness*, **29**(6), 931–954.

Griffith, C.H., Wilson, J.F., Langer, S., and Haist, S.A. (2003). House staff nonverbal communication skills and standardized patient satisfaction. *Journal of General Internal Medicine*, **18**(3), 170–174.

Guadagnoli, E. and Ward, P. (1998). Patient participation in decision-making. *Social Science and Medicine*, **47**(3), 329–339.

Gunaratnam, Y. (2001). 'We mustn't judge people . . . but': Staff dilemmas in dealing with racial harassment amongst hospice service users. *Sociology of Health and Illness*, **23**(1), 65–84.

Hagerty, R., Butow, P.N., Ellis, P.M., Lobb, E., Pendlebury, S., Leigh, N., MacLeod, C., and Tattersall, M.H. (2005). Communicating with realism and hope: Incurable cancer patients' views on the disclosure of prognosis. *Journal of Clinical Oncology*, **23**(6), 1278–1288.

Haidet, P. and Paterniti, D.A. (2003). 'Building' a history rather than 'taking' one: A perspective on information sharing during the medical interview. *Archives of Internal Medicine*, **163**(10), 1134–1140.

Hall, J.A., Harrigan, J.A., and Rosenthal, R. (1995). Nonverbal behaviour in clinician–patient interaction. *Applied and Preventive Psychology*, **4**(1), 21–35.

Hampton, J.R., Harrison, M.J., Mitchell, J.R., Prichard, J.S., and Seymour, C. (1975). Relative contributions of history-taking, physical examination, and laboratory investigation to diagnosis and management of medical outpatients. *British Medical Journal*, 2(5969), 486–489.

Hargie, O., Dickson, D., Boohan, M., and Hughes, K. (1998). A survey of communication skills training in UK schools of medicine: Present practices and prospective proposals. *Medical Education*, 32, 25–34.

Harrigan, J.A., Oxman, T.E., and Rosenthal, R. (1985). Rapport expressed through non-verbal behaviour. *Journal of Nonverbal Behaviour*, 9(2), 95–110.

Hart, C. and Chesson, R. (1998). Children as consumers. *British Medical Journal*, 316(7144), 1600–1603.

Hearing Concern (2006a). *Deaf Awareness – Terminology.* London: Hearing Concern.

Hearing Concern (2006b). *Top Ten Communication Tips to Remember When You Talk to People Who are Hard of Hearing.* London: Hearing Concern.

Henbest, R.J. and Stewart, M. (1990). Patient-centredness in the consultation. 1: A method of measurement. *Family Practice*, 6(4), 249–253.

Heritage, J., Robinson, J.D., Elliott, M.N., Beckett, M., and Wilkes, M. (2007). Reducing patients' unmet concerns in primary care: The difference one word can make. *Journal of General Internal Medicine*, 22(10), 1429–1433.

Hicks, G. (2006). *Making Contact – A Good Practice Guide: How to Involve and Communicate With a Deafblind Person.* London: Sense.

Hinchliff, S., Gott, M., and Galena, E. (2005). 'I daresay I might find it embarrassing': General practitioners' perspectives on discussing sexual health issues with lesbian and gay patients. *Health and Social Care in the Community*, 13(4), 345–353.

Hsieh, E. (2007). Interpreters as co-diagnosticians: Overlapping roles and services between providers and interpreters. *Social Science and Medicine*, 64, 924–937.

Hudelson, P. (2005). Improving patient–provider communication: Insights from interpreters. *Family Practice*, 22(3), 311–316.

Hunt, R. and Dick, S. (2008). *Serves You Right: Lesbian and Gay People's Expectations of Discrimination.* London: Stonewall.

Jenkins, V., Fallowfield, L., and Poole, K. (2001a). Are members of multidisciplinary teams in breast cancer aware of each other's informational roles? *Quality in Health Care*, 10(2), 70–75.

Jenkins, V., Fallowfield, L., and Saul, J. (2001b). Information needs of patients with cancer: Results from a large study in UK cancer centres. *British Journal of Cancer*, 84(1), 48–51.

Jensen, C. (2008). Sociology, systems and (patient) safety: Knowledge translations in health policy. *Sociology of Health and Illness*, 30(2), 309–324.

Johnson, A., Mercer, C., Erens, B., Copas, A., MacManus, S., Wellings, K., Fenton, K., Korovessis, C., Macdowall, W., Nanchahai, K., Purdon, S., and Field, J. (2001). Sexual behaviour in Britain: Partnerships, practices, and HIV risk behaviours. *The Lancet*, 358(1835), 1842.

Jurkovich, G., Pierce, B., Pananen, L., and Rivara, F. (2000). Giving bad news: The family perspective. *Journal of Trauma*, 48(5), 865–870.

Kai, J. (1999). *Valuing Diversity: A Resource for Effective Health Care of Ethnically Diverse Communities.* London: The Royal College of General Practitioners.

Kai, J., Bridgewater, R., and Spencer, J. (2006a). 'Just think of TB and Asians, that's all I ever hear': Medical learners' views about training to work in an ethnically diverse society. *Medical Education*, 35(3), 250–256.

Kai, J., Spencer, J., and Woodward, N. (2006b). Wrestling with ethnic diversity: Toward empowering health educators. *Medical Education*, 35(3), 262–271.

King, J. (1999). Giving feedback. *British Medical Journal*, 318(7200), S2.

Kirkpatrick, A. (2004). Resolving complaints. *Student British Medical Journal*, 12, 89–132.

Kirmayer, L., Groleau, D., Looper, K., and Dao, M. (2004). Explaining medically unexplained symptoms. *Canadian Journal of Psychiatry*, 49(10), 663–672.

Kleinman, A., Eisenberg, L., and Good, B. (1978). Culture, illness, and care: Clinical lessons from anthropologic and cross-cultural research. *Annals of Internal Medicine*, 88(2), 251–258.

Kneebone, R. and Nestel, D. (2005). Learning clinical skills – The place of feedback and simulation. *The Clinical Teacher*, 2(2), 86–90.

Kneebone, R., Nestel, D., Yadollah, F., Brown, R., Nolan, C., Durack, J., Brenton, H., Moulton, C., Archer, J., and Darzi, A. (2006). Assessing procedural skills in context: Exploring the feasibility of an Integrated Procedural Performance Instrument (IPPI). *Medical Education*, 40, 1105–1114.

Knox, R., Butow, P.N., Devine, R., and Tattersall, M.H. (2002). Audiotapes of oncology consultations: Only for the first consultation? *Annals of Oncology*, 13(4), 622–627.

Kohn, L., Corrigan, J., and Donaldson, M. (2000). *To Err is Human – Building a Safer Health System.* Washington, DC: Institute of Medicine, National Academy Press.

Kurtz, S., Silverman, J., Benson, J., and Draper, J. (2003). Marrying content and process in clinical method teaching: Enhancing the Calgary–Cambridge guides. *Academic Medicine*, 78(8), 802–809.

Kvalsvig, A. (2003). Ask the elephant. *The Lancet*, **362**(9401), 2079–2080.

Lanceley, A., Savage, J., Menon, U., and Jacobs, I. (2008). Influences on multidisciplinary team decision-making. *International Journal of Gynaecological Cancer*, **18**, 215–222.

Lau, F. (2000). Can communication skills workshops for emergency department doctors improve patient satisfaction? *Emergency Medicine Journal*, **17**(4), 251–253.

Lavelle-Jones, C., Byrne, D.J., Rice, P., and Cuschieri, A. (1993). Factors affecting quality of informed consent. *British Medical Journal*, **306**(6882), 885–890.

Lemos, P. and Crane, G. (2000). *Tackling Racial Harassment in the NHS: Evaluating Black and Minority Ehnic Staff's Atitudes and Experiences*. London: Department of Health.

Lewis, S. and Guthrie, E. (2002). *Master Medicine: A Clinical Core Text with Self Assessment*. Oxford: Churchill Livingstone.

Lingard, L., Garwood, K., Schryer, C., and Spafford, M. (2003). A certain art of uncertainty: Case presentation and the development of professional identity. *Social Science and Medicine*, **56**(3), 603–616.

Lutfey, K. and Freese, J. (2007). Ambiguities of chronic illness management and challenges to the medical error paradigm. *Social Science and Medicine*, **64**, 314–325.

Macdonald, E. (2004). *Difficult Conversations in Medicine*. Oxford: Oxford University Press.

Maguire, P. and Pitceathly, C. (2002). Key communication skills and how to acquire them. *British Medical Journal*, **325**(7366), 697–700.

Maguire, P., Faulkner, A., Booth, K., Elliott, C., and Hillier, V. (1996a). Helping cancer patients disclose their concerns. *European Journal of Cancer*, **32A**(1), 78–81.

Maguire, P., Booth, K., Elliott, C., and Jones, B. (1996b). Helping health professionals involved in cancer care acquire key interviewing skills–the impact of workshops. *European Journal of Cancer*, **32A**(9), 1486–1489.

Makoul, G. (2001). Essential elements of communication in medical encounters: The Kalamazoo consensus statement. *Academic Medicine*, **76**(4), 390–393.

Mangione-Smith, R., McGlynn, E.A., Elliott, M.N., McDonald, L., Franz, C.E., and Kravitz, R.L. (2001). Parent expectations for antibiotics, physician–parent communication, and satisfaction. *Archives of Pediatric and Adolescent Medicine*, **155**(7), 800–806.

Marvel, M., Epstein, R., Flowers, K., and Beckham, H. (1999). Soliciting the patient's agenda: Have we improved? *Journal of the American Medical Association*, **281**(3), 283–287.

Mayer, R., Cassel, C., Emmanuel, E., and Schnipper, L. (1998). *Report of the Task Force on End of Life Issues*. 34th Annual Meeting of the American Society of Clinical Oncology, Los Angeles: ASCO.

McCabe, R., Heath, C., Burns, T., and Priebe, S. (2002). Engagement of patients with psychosis in the consultation: Conversation analytic study. *British Medical Journal*, **325**(7373), 1148–1151.

McConnell, D., Butow, P.N., and Tattersall, M.H. (1999). Audiotapes and letters to patients: The practice and views of oncologists, surgeons and general practitioners. *British Journal of Cancer*, **79**(11/12), 1782–1788.

McDonald, P. and O'Dowd, T. (1991). The heartsink patient: A preliminary study. *Family Practice*, **8**, 112–116.

McGee, S. and Irby, D. (1997). Teaching in the outpatient clinic: Practical tips. *Journal of General Internal Medicine*, **12**(S2), S34–S40.

McGrath, P. and Huff, N. (2001). 'What is it?': Findings on preschoolers' responses to play with medical equipment. *Child: Care, Health and Development*, **27**(5), 451–462.

McKelvey, R., Webb, J., Baldassar, L., Robinson, S., and Riley, G. (1999). Sex knowledge and sexual attitudes among medical and nursing students. *Australian and New Zealand Journal of Psychiatry*, **33**, 260–266.

McKinley, R.K. and Middleton, J.F. (1999). What do patients want from doctors? Content analysis of written patient agendas for the consultation. *British Journal of General Practice*, **49**(447), 796–800.

Medical Protection Society (2008). *MPS Guide to Medical Records*. London: Medical Protection Society.

Miller, P., Parker, S., and Gillinson, S. (2004). *Disablism: How to Tackle the Last Prejudice*. London: Demos.

Miner, H. (1956). Body ritual among the Nacirema. *American Anthropologist*, **58**(3), 503–507.

Mitchell, P. and Zeigler, F. (2007). *Fundamentals of Development: The Psychology of Childhood*. Hove: Psychology Press.

Moss, B. and Roberts, C. (2005). Explanations, explanations, explanations: How do patients with limited English construct narrative accounts in multi-lingual, multi-ethnic settings, and how can GPs interpret them? *Family Practice*, **22**(4), 412–418.

Mumford, E., Schlesinger, H.J., and Glass, G.V. (1982). The effect of psychological intervention on recovery from surgery and heart attacks: An analysis of the literature. *American Journal of Public Health*, **72**(2), 141–151.

Munro, D., Bore, M., and Powis, D. (2005). Personality factors in professional ethical behaviour: Studies of empathy and narcissism. *Australian Journal of Psychology*, **57**(1), 49–60.

National Institute on Deafness and Other Communication Disorders (1997). *Aphasia*. Bethesda, MD, USA: National Institute on Deafness and Other Communication Disorders.

National Patient Safety Agency (2005). *Being Open When Patients Are Harmed*. London: National Patient Safety Agency.

Ngo-Metzger, Q., Massagli, M.P., Clarridge, B.R., Manocchia, M., Davis, R.B., Iezzoni, L.I., and Phillips, R.S. (2003). Linguistic and cultural barriers to care. *Journal of General Internal Medicine*, **18**(1), 44–52.

NHS Litigation Authority (2007). *Apologies and Explanations*. London: NHS Litigation Authority.

Noble, L. (2007). Written communication. In: S. Ayers, A. Baum, C. McManus, S. Newman, K. Wallston, J. Weinman, and R. West (Eds), *Cambridge Handbook of Psychology, Health and Medicine*. Cambridge: Cambridge University Press, pp. 517–521.

North London Cancer Network (2006). *Communicating Significant News*. London: North London Cancer Care Network.

O'Connor, A.M., Rostom, A., Fiset, V., Tetroe, J., Entwistle, V., Llewellyn-Thomas, H., Holmes-Rovner, M., Barry, M., and Jones, J. (1999). Decision aids for patients facing health treatment or screening decisions: Systematic review. *British Medical Journal*, **319**(7212), 731–734.

O'Dowd, T. (1988). Five years of heartsink patients in general practice. *British Medical Journal*, **297**, 528.

Office of National Statistics (2001). *Psychiatric Morbidity Among Adults Living in Private Households*. London: HMSO.

Parker, P., Baile, W.F., de Moor, C., Lenzi, R., Kudelka, A.P., and Cohen, L. (2001). Breaking bad news about cancer: Patients' preferences for communication. *Journal of Clinical Oncology*, **19**(7), 2049–2056.

Pendleton, D., Schofield, T., Tate, P., and Havelock, P. (1984). *The Consultation: An Approach to Learning and Teaching*. Oxford: Oxford University Press.

Perrin, E.C. and Gerrity, P.S. (1981). There's a demon in your belly: Children's understanding of illness. *Pediatrics*, **67**(6), 841–849.

Perry, J. (1994). Communicating with toddlers in hospital. *Paediatric Nursing*, **6**(5), 14–17.

Peterson, M.C., Holbrook, J., VonHales, D., Smith, N.L., and Staker, L.V. (1992). Contributions of the history, physical examination and laboratory investigation in making medical diagnoses. *Western Journal of Medicine*, **156**(2), 163–165.

Phitayakorn, R., Williams, R., Yudkowsky, R., Harris, I., Hauge, L., Widmann, W., Sullivan, M., and Mellinger, J. (2008). Patient-care-related telephone communication between general surgery residents and attending surgeons. *Journal of the American College of Surgeons*, **206**(4), 742–750.

Pinnock, H., Bawden, R., Proctor, S., Wolfe, S., Scullion, J., Price, D., and Sheikh, A. (2003). Accessibility, acceptability, and effectiveness in primary care of routine telephone review of asthma: Pragmatic, randomised controlled trial. *British Medical Journal*, **326**(7387), 477–479.

Porter, J., Ouvry, C., Morgan, M., and Downs, C. (2001). Interpreting the communication of people with profound and multiple learning difficulties. *British Journal of Learning Disabilities*, **29**, 12–16.

Prkachin, K. and Craig, K. (1995). Expressing pain: The communication and interpretation of facial pain signals. *Journal of Nonverbal Behaviour*, **19**(4), 191–205.

Ramirez, A., Graham, J., Richards, M., Cull, A., and Gregory, W. (1996). Mental health of hospital consultants: The effects of stress and satisfaction at work. *The Lancet*, **347**, 724–728.

Regnard, C., Reynolds, J., Watson, B., Matthews, D., Gibson, L., and Clarke, C. (2007). Understanding distress in people with severe communication difficulties: Developing and assessing the Disability Distress Assessment Tool (DisDAT). *Journal of Intellectual Disability Research*, **51**(4), 277–292.

Rhoades, D.R., McFarland, K.F., Finch, W.H., and Johnson, A.O. (2001). Speaking and interruptions during primary care office visits. *Family Medicine*, **33**(7), 528–532.

Risdon, C., Cook, D., and Willms, D. (2000). Gay and lesbian physicians in training: A qualitative study. *Canadian Medical Association Journal*, **162**(3), 331–334.

RNID (2006). Communication tips for hearing people. London: Royal National Institute of the Deaf.

Robinson, J.D. (2001). Closing medical encounters: Two physician practices and their implications for the expression of patients' unstated concerns. *Social Science and Medicine*, **53**(5), 639–656.

Rose, L. (1994). Homophobia among doctors. *British Medical Journal*, **308**(6928), 586–587.

Rosen, R., and Dewar, S. (2004). *On Being a Doctor: Redefining Medical Professionalism for Better Patient Care*. London: Kings Fund.

Rosendal, M., Fink, P., Bro, F., and Olesen, F. (2005). Somatization, heartsink patients, or functional somatic symptoms? Towards a clinical useful classification in primary health care. *Scandinavian Journal of Primary Health Care*, **23**, 3–10.

RSM Forum on Communication in Healthcare (2004). Core curriculum for communication skills learning in medical schools. In: E. McDonald (Ed.), *Difficult Conversations in Medicine*, Oxford: Oxford University Press, 209–211.

Ruusuvuori, J. (2001). Looking means listening: Coordinating displays of engagement in doctor–patient interaction. *Social Science and Medicine*, **52**(7), 1093–1108.

Salmon, P., Peters, S., and Stanley, I. (1999). Patients' perceptions of medical explanations for somatisation disorders: Qualitative analysis. *British Medical Journal*, **318**(7180), 372–376.

Salmon, P., Ring, A., Dowrick, C., and Humphris, G. (2005). What do general practice patients want when they present medically unexplained symptoms, and why do their doctors feel pressurized? *Journal of Psychosomatic Research*, **59**, 255–262.

Sanders, T. and Harrison, S. (2008). Professional legitimacy claims in the multidisciplinary workplace: The case of heart failure care. *Sociology of Health and Illness*, **30**(2), 289–308.

Schildmann, J., Cushing, A., Doyal, L., and Vollmann, J. (2005). Breaking bad news: Experiences, views and difficulties of pre-registration house officers. *Palliative Medicine*, **19**(2), 93–98.

Schouten, B.C. and Meeuwesen, L. (2006). Cultural differences in medical communication: A review of the literature. *Patient Education and Counselling*, **64**, 21–34.

Scott, J.T., Entwistle, V.A., Sowden, A.J., and Watt, I. (2001). Giving tape recordings or written summaries of consultations to people with cancer: A systematic review. *Health Expectations*, **4**(3), 162–169.

Sense (2003). *How Do People Who Are Deafblind Communicate?* London: Sense.

Sense (2006). *Communicating With Your Deafblind Patients.* London: Sense.

Sense About Science (2008). *Making Sense of Testing: A Guide to Why Scans and Health Tests For Well People Aren't Aways a Good Idea.* London: Sense About Science.

Sense and Deafblind UK (2001). *Who Cares? Access to Healthcare for Deafblind People.* London: Sense and Deafblind UK.

Sexton, J., Thomas, E., and Helmreich, R. (2000). Error, stress, and teamwork in medicine and aviation: Cross sectional surveys. *British Medical Journal*, **320**(7237), 745–749.

Shapiro, R. (2008). *Suckers: How Alternative Medicine Makes Fools of Us All.* London: Harvill Secker.

Shohet, R. (2005). *Passionate Medicine: Making the Transition From Conventional Medicine to Homeopathy.* London and Philadelphia: Jessica Kingsley Publishers.

Shorter, E. (1992). *From Paralysis to Fatigue: A History of Psychosomatic Illness in the Modern Era.* New York: The Free Press.

Showalter, E. (1997). *Hystories: Hysterical Epidemics and Modern Media.* New York: Columbia University Press.

Silverman, J., Kurtz, S., and Draper, J. (2005). *Skills for Communicating with Patients*, 2nd edn. Oxford: Radcliffe Medical Press.

Simpson, M., Buckman, R., Stewart, M., Maguire, P., Lipkin, M., Novack, D., and Till, J. (1991). Doctor–patient communication: The Toronto consensus statement. *British Medical Journal*, **303**(6814), 1385–1387.

Singh, S. and Ernst, E. (2008). *Trick or Treatment: Alternative Medicine on Trial.* London: Bantam Press.

Smith, G., Bartlett, A., and King, M. (2004). Treatments of homosexuality in Britain since the 1950s – An oral history: The experience of patients. *British Medical Journal*, **328**(7437), 427.

Sontag, S. (1978). *Illness as Metaphor.* London: Penguin Books.

Sontag, S. (1989). *AIDS and its Metaphors.* USA: Farra, Straus & Giroux.

Spiro, H. (1992). What is empathy and can it be taught? *Annals of Internal Medicine*, **116**(10), 843–846.

Stacey, D., Hawker, G., Dervin, G., Tomek, I., Cochran, N., Tugwell, P., and O'Connor, A.M. (2008). Improving shared decision making in osteoarthritis. *British Medical Journal*, **336**(650), 954–955.

Stephenson, A., Higgs, R., and Sugarman, J. (2001). Teaching professional development in medical schools. *The Lancet*, **357**, 867–870.

Stevenson, F.A., Barry, C.A., Britten, N., Barber, N., and Bradley, C.P. (2000). Doctor–patient communication about drugs: The evidence for shared decision making. *Social Science and Medicine*, **50**(6), 829–840.

Stewart, M. (2001). Towards a global definition of patient centred care. *British Medical Journal*, **322**(7284), 444–4445.

Stockl, A. (2007). Complex syndromes, ambivalent diagnosis, and existential uncertainty: The case of Systemic Lupus Erythematosus (SLE). *Social Science and Medicine*, **65**, 1549–1559.

Stringer, S., Church, L., Davidson, S. and Lipsedge, M. (Eds) (2009). *Psychiatry PRN: Principles, Reality, Next Steps.* Oxford: Oxford University Press.

Suchman, A.L. (2003). Research on patient–clinician relationships: Celebrating success and identifying the next scope of work. *Journal of General Internal Medicine*, **18**(8), 677–678.

Surbone, A. (2008). Cultural aspects of communication in cancer care. *Support Cancer Care*, **16**, 235–240.

Tate, P. (2005). Ideas, concerns and expectations. *Medicine*, **33**(2), 26–27.

Tates, K. and Meeuwesen, L. (2000). 'Let mum have her say': Turntaking in doctor–parent–child communication. *Patient Education and Counselling*, **40**(2), 151–162.

Taylor-Adams, S., Vincent, C., and Stanhope, N. (1999). Applying human factors methods to the investigation and analysis of clinical adverse events. *Safety Science*, **31**, 143–159.

Tesser, A., Rosen, S., and Tesser, M. (1971). On the reluctance to communicate undesirable messages (the MUM effect). A field study. *Psychological Reports*, **29**, 651–654.

The Disability Partnership (2000). *One in Four of Us: The Experience of Disability*. London: The Disability Partnership.

The Headache Study Group of The University of Western Ontario (1986). Predictors of outcome in headache patients presenting to family physicians. A one year prospective study. *Headache: The Journal of Head and Face Pain*, **26**(6), 285–294.

Thomson, R., Edwards, A., and Grey, J. (2005). Risk communication in the clinical consultation. *Clinical Medicine*, **5**(5), 465–469.

Thornton, H., Edwards, A., and Baum, M. (2003). Women need better information about routine mammography. *British Medical Journal*, **327**(7406), 101–103.

Thurman, S., Jones, J., and Tarleton, B. (2005). Without words – meaningful information for people with high individual communication needs. *British Journal of Learning Disabilities*, **33**, 83–89.

Tomlinson, J. (1998). ABC of sexual health: Taking a sexual history. *British Medical Journal*, **317**(7172), 1573–1576.

Toon, P.D. (2002). Using telephones in primary care. *British Medical Journal*, **324**(7348), 1230–1231.

Tovey, P. and Broom, A. (2007). Oncologists' and specialist cancer nurses' approaches to complemetary and alternative medicine and their impact on patient action. *Social Science and Medicine*, **64**, 2550–2564.

Turner, K., Ireland, L., Krenus, B., and Pointon, L. (2007). *Essential Academic Skills*. Oxford: Oxford University Press.

Vincent, C., Stanhope, N., and Crowley-Murphey, M. (1999). Reasons for not reporting adverse events: An empirical study. *Journal of Evaluation in Clinical Practice*, **5**(1), 13–21.

Vincent, C., Neale, G., and Woloshynowych, M. (2001). Adverse events in British hospitals: Preliminary retrospective record review. *British Medical Journal*, **322**(7285), 517–519.

Verhoeven, V., Bovijn, K., Helder, A., Peremans, L., Hermann, I., van Royen, P., Deenkens, J., and Avonts, D. (2003). Discussing STIs: Doctors are from Mars, patients from Venus. *Family Practice*, **20**(1), 11–15.

Vincent, C., Young, A., and Phillips, A. (1994). Why do patients sue doctors? A study of patients and relatives taking legal action. *The Lancet*, **343**(8913), 1609–1613.

von Fragstein, M., Silverman, J., Cushing, A., Quilligan, S., Salisbury, H., and Wiskin, C. (2008). UK consensus statement on the content of communication curricula in undergraduate medical education. *Medical Education* **42**(11), 1100–1107.

von Gunten, C., Ferris, F., and Emanuel, L. (2000). Ensuring competency in end-of-life care: Communication and relational skills. *Journal of the American Medical Association*, **284**(23), 3051–3057.

Waitzkin, H. (1985). Information giving in medical care. *Journal of Health and Social Behavior*, **26**(2), 81–101.

Wallace, J. and Lemaire, J. (2007). On physician well being – You'll get by with a little help from your friends. *Social Science & Medicine*, **64**, 2565–2577.

Waring, J. (2005). Beyond blame: Cultural barriers to medical incident reporting. *Social Science and Medicine*, **60**, 1927–1935.

Warner, J., McKeown, E., Griffin, M., Johnson, K., Ramsay, A., Cort, C., and King, M. (2004). Rates and predictors of mental illness in gay men, lesbians and bisexual men and women: Results from a survey based in England and Wales. *The British Journal of Psychiatry*, **185**(6), 479–485.

Weiner, B., Hobgood, C., and Lewis, M. (2008). The meaning of justice in safety incident reporting. *Social Science and Medicine*, **66**, 403–413.

Westerstahl, A., Segesten, K., and Bjorkelund, C. (2002). GPs and lesbian women in the consultation: Issues of awareness and knowledge. *Scandinavian Journal of Primary Health Care*, **20**(4), 203–207.

White, C. (2004a). Doctors mistrust systems for reporting medical mistakes. *British Medical Journal*, **329**(7456), 12–13.

White, P. (2004b). Copying referral letters to patients: Prepare for change. *Patient Education and Counselling*, **54**(2), 159–161.

White, J.C., Rosson, C., Christensen, J., Hart, R., and Levinson, W. (1997). Wrapping things up: A qualitative analysis of the closing moments of the medical visit. *Patient Education and Counselling*, **30**(2), 155–165.

WHO (2002). *Sexual Health*. Geneva: The World Health Organization.

Williams, S., Dale, J., Glucksman, E., and Wellesley, A. (1997). Senior house officers' work related stressors, psychological distress, and confidence in performing clinical tasks in accident and emergency: A questionnaire study. *British Medical Journal*, **314**(7082), 713–718.

Windebank, K. and Spinetta, J. (2008). Do as I say or die: Compliance in adolescents with cancer. *Pediatric Blood Cancer*, **50**, 1099–1100.

Wittenberg-Lyles, E., Goldsmith, J., Sanchez-Reilly, S., and Ragan, S. (2008). Communicating a terminal prognosis in a palliative care setting: Deficiencies in current communication training protocols. *Social Science & Medicine*, **66**, 2356–2365.

Woloshin, S., Schwartz, L., and Ellner, A. (2003). Making sense of risk information on the web: Don't forget the basics. *British Medical Journal*, **327**(7417), 695–696.

Woolf, K. and Kavanagh, J. (2006). Giving presentations without palpitations. *British Medical Journal Careers Focus*, **332**, 242–243.

Zollman, C. and Vickers, C. (1999a). ABC of complementary medicine: Complementary medicine and the patient. *British Medical Journal*, **319**(7223), 1486–1489.

Zollman, C. and Vickers, C. (1999b). ABC of complementary medicine: Complementary medicine and the doctor. *British Medical Journal*, **319**(7224), 1558–1561.

Index